VITAMIN E, ANYONE?

"Though it was first discovered a half-century ago, Vitamin E has long been pretty much of a mystery to medical men . . . There is no question that it is a vital nutrient . . . In recent months, Vitamin E has become something of a cult . . . The demand for Vitamin E pills is soaring. In some areas, pharmacies and health-food stores report sales of the vitamin up by 500 percent compared with a year ago . . .

"One of the foremost advocates of Vitamin E is Dr. Evan V. Shute, head of the Shute Institute for Clinical and Laboratory Medicine in London, Ontario. 'It's the most versatile vitamin,' the Canadian doctor said. 'It provides better circulation and oxygenation and enhances the power of the muscles. Almost nothing in the body wouldn't be improved by a large intake of Vitamin E.'"

—Newsweek

THE TRUTH ABOUT VITAMIN E

Acknowledgments

The author of this volume is indebted to the helpful informational assistance of The Shute Foundation, The Nutrition Foundation, the Vitamin Information Service, the Food and Agricultural Development Laboratory of Hoffman-LaRoche, Inc., and to the Distillation Products Industries division of the Eastman Kodak Company; details on these and other sources may be found in the *Selected Bibliography* (pp. 144-149).

A work such as this must of necessity be the product of research and writing by more than a single individual. The author gratefully acknowledges the help of William R. Akins and Helen McCarthy, as well as of his colleagues at Lombard Associates, Inc., notably Michael Ballantine, George Mavros, and Pamela White.

THE TRUTH
ABOUT VITAMIN E

Martin Ebon

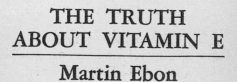

A NATIONAL GENERAL COMPANY

THE TRUTH ABOUT VITAMIN E

A Bantam Book / published July 1972

Library of Congress Cataloging in Publication Data

Ebon, Martin.
    The truth about vitamin E.

    Bibliography: p.
    1. Tocopherol. I. Title.
RM666.T65E26   615'.328   72-3006

Published simultaneously in the United States and Canada

Bantam Books are published by Bantam Books, Inc., a National
General company. Its trade-mark, consisting of the words "Bantam
Books" and the portrayal of a bantam, is registered in the United
States Patent Office and in other countries. Marca Registrada.
Bantam Books, Inc., 666 Fifth Avenue, New York, N.Y. 10019.

PRINTED IN THE UNITED STATES OF AMERICA

Table of Contents

ture Birth—Vitamin E and Infant Disease
—Vitamin E and Birth Defects—Danger
of Toxemia—Preparing for Pregnancy 76

1   Vitamin E: What It Is,
What It Does

What exactly is Vitamin E? What are its unique medical uses, to heal or to prevent disease? Can Vitamin E help you improve your personal well-being?

These are the basic questions this book sets out to answer.

In phrasing our answers, we shall be straightforward as well as cautious. Vitamin E is a center of controversy. One reason for this is that nutritional and medical research into its properties is quite new. Another is the fact that exaggerated claims and medical caution clash head-on when it comes to Vitamin E. We will try to steer a middle course between overenthusiasm and ultra-conservatism.

Vitamin E was first discovered in the early 1920s, by Drs. Herbert M. Evans and Katherine S. Bishop. They found that experimental animals that lacked this vitamin lost their sexual capacities. This discovery helped give Vitamin E the label of the "antisterility" vitamin. During the past half-century these findings have been reinforced by numerous additional experiments.

Perhaps the most striking quality of Vitamin E lies in its effect on the blood. Experiments have shown that the vitamin is involved in the blood to the extent that it affects just about everything from circulation to heart functioning. Precisely how these most essential functions are performed no one really knows. It always amazes nonmedical people that, often in essential areas, medical science frequently does not know how a particular substance or treatment can effect a cure. No one actually knows exactly how aspirin works. And something that fulfills such complex functions as Vitamin E is even more mysterious. One reason for this is the relation of E to other vitamins in the body; the other is that there is no feasible scientific way to test it.

Instead, we have to rely on indirect findings. For example, the work done recently by two physicians in Wales, Drs. M. A. Chadd and A. J. Fraser, throws light on the role of Vitamin E in combating anemia (the condition laymen call "thinning" of the blood which occurs when the number of red blood cells decreases to a danger point). Drs. Chadd and Fraser studied fifty-two babies of varying weight, some of whom were given Vitamin E supplements. Regardless of weight, all the babies given the vitamin had higher blood levels of Vitamin E within a week, which showed that they absorbed the vitamin quite easily. And at the crucial point when newborn infants might develop anemia, the Vitamin E babies showed a higher blood level than those who had not received the supplement.

The report of the two doctors, which appeared in the *International Journal of Vitamin Research,* takes into account that most babies are born with a vitamin deficiency, because Vitamin E does not pass from the pregnant mother to the baby. Usually this deficiency is made up within a few weeks, particularly if the baby is breast fed. But premature babies and newborn infants who are severely underweight at times suffer anemia that does not respond to

2

the common iron supplements. That is why the Vitamin E treatment may literally save the lives of premature and underweight babies. Some baby formulas are high in unsaturated fats. This makes additional Vitamin E even more essential, because this vitamin is needed for these fats to be broken down and utilized properly by the body.

In a later article in the same research journal, the two Welsh doctors reported on three babies who had been born "grossly premature." They were anemic and their bodies were swollen. Routine vitamin supplements, iron and folic acid—which is a B vitamin—had not helped them. But when the doctors gave them twelve milligrams of Vitamin E, their swellings went down immediately and the red blood cells increased in number. Drs. Chadd and Fraser suggest that doctors treating "any small infant who has an anemia within a few weeks of birth" should consider that the baby may be suffering from a Vitamin E deficiency.

The U.S. magazine *Better Nutrition* (August 1971) illustrated the Vitamin E dilemma well when it commented on the findings of these two Welsh doctors. It speculated that the mothers of the babies may themselves have been lacking Vitamin E in their diet. The magazine asked, "But if the vitamin E does not pass readily from mother to unborn child, does it not seem possible that this may be because of lack of vitamin E in the mother? Many researchers have shown that modern diets in which refined foods make up a large part are lacking in this vitamin. Is it not possible that these infants' mothers were just not getting enough of it to pass along to the babies?"

The magazine then poses this question: "Considering the close relationship of vitamin E to reproductive functions, isn't it possible, too, that lack of vitamin E in the mother's diet may be one of the main reasons for the babies being born prematurely?" A challenging question.

3

But so far medical research can only make this one-word reply: "Perhaps." Lack of Vitamin E has caused insufficient embryo development, as well as sterility in male laboratory animals (rats and mice). There is only one step from unsatisfactory embryo growth to premature birth, but factors other than Vitamin E deficiency may be involved.

We don't want you to be impatient with the medical profession when you read about Vitamin E. While its uses were first defined in the 1920s, extensive research has taken place only during the last couple of decades. And while we may assume that what is true for rats and rabbits is likely to be true for people, at least where vitamin needs are concerned, there are enough gaps in our knowledge to preclude our saying, for instance, "Yes, of course, the mothers of these preemies were probably lacking in Vitamin E."

Pregnant mothers and breast-feeding mothers do need Vitamin E. There is simply no doubt about that. And while we do not advocate self-medication, we also know that crucial vitamins are lacking in much of our everyday food; in the case of Vitamin E supplements are necessary. One leading specialist, Dr. David Herting, has said that physicians and nutritionists are concerned with the "danger of a marginal deficiency or gradual depletion which does not show any immediate overt signs or which is obscured by other dietary or environmental factors."

How Safe Is Vitamin E?

Before we go any further you may well ask, "How safe is Vitamin E?" We wish you could get all the Vitamin E you needed by simply eating whole grain cereals or nuts or olives in sufficient quantity. But unfortunately this is not possible. And we cannot even castigate the food processor for robbing us of essential vitamins. We simply have to recognize these deficiencies and try to make up for them. As Dr. Herting points out, you may suffer from a Vitamin E deficiency and not know it—because your symptoms are too slight to be noticed; you may ascribe them to job problems, family difficulties, or to some hereditary condition. But you never know.

Still, the question remains: Is Vitamin E safe? Of course, you should not go on any nutritional binges. They don't last, anyhow. Self-medication is not recommended and doses should respond to individual needs. Even though a background memorandum of the Vitamin Information Office notes that "possible harm produced by vitamin E *excess* has not yet been demonstrated in man or animals," any chemical agent strong enough to aid can do harm in an overdose—unless it is Vitamin C, which the body eliminates quickly.

Vitamin E does not stand alone. Its actions within the human body are closely related to its better known cousin, Vitamin C. Both vitamins help the blood absorb essential iron; both are highly concentrated in the adrenal gland, which controls much of body chemistry; and some experimental animals have shown that Vitamin E is necessary for the normal integration of Vitamin C.

Vitamin E is usually given in the form of an oval capsule that shows a light golden-yellow liquid. Back in 1936 it was first isolated from wheat germ oil. Its technical name since then has been *tocopherol;* the word is made up from the Greek *tokos* (childbirth) and *pherein* (to bear), a reference to Vitamin E's relation to fertility. There are four major types of tocopherol. Of these, alpha-tocopherol is of the greatest nutritional importance. Tocopherol is mainly stored in the liver and fatty tissues of the body. Dr. Herting has said that the thousands of investigations into Vitamin E deficiency have shown perhaps "the largest variety of disorders associated with the nutritional deficiency of any single vitamin."

Keeping the Doctor Away

One can deduce from Dr. Herting's statement that Vitamin E can help eliminate more deficiencies than any other vitamin. That means, of course, by turning the negative side—that lack of Vitamin E creates symptoms of disease—into the positive finding that the use of Vitamin E can prevent or roll back disease. We are for preventive medicine ourselves; we favor well-rounded nutrition that helps avoid deficiencies and disease. An apple a day may not keep the doctor away, and neither may Vitamin E (together with other selected nutritional elements), but they can make visits to the doctor less frequent or necessary.

We have seen part of the role that Vitamin E plays in counteracting anemia in newborn babies. At the other end of the spectrum, in the area of human aging, it appears to have significance in holding back arteriosclerosis, the so-called hardening of the arteries. The accumulation of solid matter inside the arteries, which eventually narrows them dangerously, begins to occur at an early age. Children are thus developing narrowed arterial canals. The process seems to be irreversible. To the degree that Vitamin E can reduce these deposits, it delays the aging process and literally prolongs life.

Experiments also point to the role of Vitamin E in counteracting protein deficiencies. This is a vast field, because many parts of the body need the constant intake of properly absorbable protein. It has been shown in experimental animals that lack of Vitamin E may be linked

6

with liver necrosis (disintegration of the liver). One of the most striking discoveries has occurred in one of the most dramatic diseases of our time, muscular dystrophy. Vitamin E counteracts nutritional muscular dystrophy in animals, even monkeys, but cannot be used against muscular dystrophy in humans.

Perhaps the widest area of Vitamin E deficiency among adults in the United States is in gastrointestinal disease. Prolonged Vitamin E deficiency can cause faulty absorption of fat and of fat-soluble vitamins. Cystic fibrosis, blockage of the bile duct, and chronic inflammation of the pancreas are among the disorders that can result, at least theoretically.

Thus we see that the body's need for Vitamin E ranges widely. This has created, for researchers and medical practitioners, an embarrassment of riches. Vitamin E cannot be type cast. The editors of the *New England Journal of Medicine* have written, with a mixture of awe and curiosity, that "the diversity of pathological conditions in which deficiency of the vitamin is thought to be involved confounds, rather than illuminates, its metabolic properties." This just means that Vitamin E can do you a lot of good, in a lot of different ways. On the following pages we will try to show you how Vitamin E can help restore the nutritional balance of your body that modern food processing has thrown out of kilter.

II Keeping Your Blood Young

Heart and circulatory diseases show a very definite geographical distribution, probably caused by the varying diets around the world. These particular diseases are highest in the United States, second highest in Britain, and third highest in Scotland and Switzerland. As the famous American authority on Chinese medicine Dr. Isidor Snapper has noted, cardiovascular-renal heart disease is very much less in evidence in China. The rarity of heart attacks due to blood clotting, as well as angina pectoris and arteriosclerosis, is particularly striking as its rate of increase in the United States continues to soar.

Dr. Snapper notes that hardening of the arteries is seldom encountered in the autopsies of middle-aged Chinese, whereas it is frequently found in the autopsies of even young Americans. He believes that these geographical differences in heart and blood pathology are best explained by differences in nutrition. He points out that the Chinese have lower blood pressure and that their fat intake is considerably different from that of Americans. The Chinese diet is quite different from the American diet of butter and other dairy products rich in cholesterol. The Chinese diet is naturally rich in Vitamin E; the Chinese use sesame oil, peanut oil, or soybean oil for frying their

8

foods, and thus not only receive a substantially larger intake of Vitamin E but, over a lifetime, consume large amounts of linoleic acid, an essential fatty acid. Both are present in limited amounts in the standard American diet.

Against Blood Clots

The main contribution of Vitamin E to the bloodstream relates to the phenomenon of clotting. If blood did not clot as a natural process, wounds, surgery, even minor injuries would all cause fatal bleeding. However, when the blood forms clots too easily (thrombosis), the results are often just as fatal. The Vitamin Information Bureau of New York City identifies Vitamin E as "necessary for normal development and functioning of red blood, muscle, cells, and other tissues." The Bureau states that the vitamin also protects tissue fat substances from abnormal breakdown and that the Vitamin E requirement "appears to vary with the amount of unsaturated fatty acid in the diet." In the absence of Vitamin E, the breakdown of cells in the blood vessels may cause clots to form. Phlebitis, inflammation of the walls of the veins, is a very common example of this.

The importance of the blood as a purveyor of health—and of illness—can hardly be overstated. The body depends upon the blood's circulation for its nourishment. A good diet, with a sufficient supplement of Vitamin E, will provide most people with blood that is nutritionally rich and circulating freely in the body; health and youthful vigor will be their inevitable rewards. On the other hand, on days when one eats poorly, one not only feels older, one actually is older biologically.

As an example of the importance of healthy food, let us consider for the moment the human need for food proteins. From the moment of our birth to that of death proteins are continuously being broken down by enzymes, and for us to survive, amino acids must be available to replace them immediately. Our bodies are composed largely of proteins, but unlike plants we cannot make our own proteins. When we eat protein foods, our digestive system breaks them down into amino acids, and these in turn pass into our blood and are carried throughout the body. The body cells select from the twenty-two amino acids those they need, and from these they construct new body tissue, as well as new blood cells. Clearly, keeping the blood young, fresh, and vital is the first step toward overall good health.

Since the circulatory system plays such an important part in supplying the body with the nutrition it needs to survive, the role of Vitamin E in providing for good health can scarcely be overlooked. Although some of its other functions may attract wider attention, the real value of Vitamin E may perhaps be that it is the main natural anti-clotting agent.

Vitamin E and Blood Vessels

After treating 166 patients who suffered from chronic phlebitis, Dr. Evan Shute found that Vitamin E therapy produced successful results in 111 cases. He also noted that Vitamin E "decreases embolism [blood clot] to the merest minimum. It not only prevents extension of existing clots, as do the classical anti-coagulants, but it quickly dissolves what clot is present. It acts very rapidly, especially in relieving associated pain and tenderness. It has none of the side effects which plague the anti-coagulants since it never produces hemorrhages, for example. Moreover, it does not require frequent blood examinations, can be self-administered far from any hospital, or even medical care, and is as useful for clots in the vital organs as for clots in the peripheral vessels." He regards it as "the only safe and cheap fibriolysis."

Still another key to the feeling of rejuvenation and youthfulness that daily doses of Vitamin E can produce is provided by Carlson Wade. He writes that the new-found energy that Vitamin E users experience is "largely depended upon a special natural blood substance known as *heparin* which is made in the liver. Heparin maintains a healthy bloodstream and also helps prevent blood coagulation." He notes that tests have found that Vitamin E was able to promote and actually *duplicate* any deficiency of heparin.

The second major effect of Vitamin E on the circulatory system is the dilation of the blood vessels. Even when the blood itself is free of clots that slow down its movements, the veins and arteries themselves must be large enough to permit the blood to pass easily. In helping to prevent slow circulation and vascular aging, Vitamin E also reduces the likelihood of cerebral strokes, coronary thrombosis, perhaps varicose veins, and related illnesses.

Diseases of the blood vessels in the leg and foot or arm and hand occur when these extremities receive a reduced supply of blood because of some abnormality in the blood vessels. Cramps and muscle spasms, phlebitis, Buerger's Disease, and arteriosclerosis are among the more common such ailments. The root difficulty lies usually in a narrowing of the bore of the blood vessel, through which the blood must flow. This condition is not uncommon with heavy smokers, who thus diminish still further the amount of blood oxygen that their bodies receive.

Writing of his patients suffering from a shrinking of the blood vessels in their arms and legs, Wilfrid Shute observed that "Alpha-tocopherol [Vitamin E] led to healing of the lesions and a partial return of pulsation to the vessels," which provided "visual evidence of the tissue-sparing action" of Vitamin E.

Oxygen in the Blood

The third major effect of Vitamin E on the circulatory system is to preserve and lessen the amount of oxygen in the bloodstream. Provided the Vitamin E intake is sufficient each day, the average life expectancy of red corpuscles is three to four months. Vitamin E may substantially lessen the need of the heart, lungs, brain, and other organs for oxygen. Premature aging and degenerative diseases of the cellular tissues are caused by insufficient oxygen and nutrients. By combining with unsaturated fatty acids, Vitamin E prevents these acids from combining with oxygen and producing age plaques (toxic peroxides and hydrocarbons) in the metabolism. By leaving the oxygen free, the blood is able to maintain a high oxygen content and to circulate it freely to all the body cells.

Obviously, not only the percentage of oxygen in the bloodstream, but also the life expectancy of the red cells, is crucial. Experimenting with hemoglobin, which carries the oxygen in the blood to the various cells and tissues, Drs. S. Luczak and F. Wolk, writing in *Deutsche Medizinische Monatsschrift*, concluded that Vitamin E helps to prolong the life of the hemoglobin so that cellular degeneration of blood vessels and tissues in the extremities is reduced. As Vitamin E is able to enhance efficiency of the blood by preserving its oxygen content, it could also aid in the repair of damaged and diseased tissues, bringing new life to them, especially those of the heart.

By reducing the fat content of the blood, not only does Vitamin E help prevent such problems of aging as heart attacks and hardening of the arteries, but its youth-giving powers also affect the whole body. Not until we are older or have fallen into ill health do we realize how much our health rested upon many things we take for granted, such as the circulation of our blood. By maintaining a high percentage of oxygen in the hemoglobin through daily intake of Vitamin E, the blood saves the heart and other organs from working overtime. When the blood is healthy, it functions more efficiently, less of it is needed by the body, hence the heart needs to pump less in order to achieve its results. With the increased preservation of blood oxygen as a result of sufficient Vitamin E, the blood is able to nourish the body's cells and tissues, preventing the degeneration of the reproductive and other organs and actually delaying the biological aging process.

What Is Aging?

From a biologic standpoint, we have limited knowledge of the aging process, but there seems little doubt that through its action on the circulatory system, Vitamin E has the power to slow down the effects of aging. Of course, the general biologic process extends over our entire lifespan. The aging process is largely conditioned by the body's consumption of Vitamin E, and other nutrients during growth and maturity. In later years, there is a loss of cells and a reduction in cell metabolism. From the age of thirty to ninety, there is a gradual decay in the performance level of most organs. For example, the speed of conducting a nerve impulse lessens by 15 percent; the rate of the blood flow through the kidney is reduced 65 percent; the heart output is reduced by 30 percent; the functional efficiency of the lungs drops by 60 per cent. And there is a reduced recovery after illness. Further

13

symptoms of age in the heart and lungs are that the pulse rate and respiration after exercise or other exertion take longer to return to normal.

The overall biologic process of aging is very closely related to nutrition, and specifically to Vitamin E. The body's reserve capacities are gradually reduced because of a loss of cell tissue. This loss is in part the result of the blood's lowered oxygen content. For people of advancing age, a daily concentrated dosage of Vitamin E becomes necessary because they may not be able to get a sufficient supply from natural foods. With age, there seems to be a diminished secretion of digestive juices, a decrease in the function of the gastrointestinal tract, as well as decreased ability to absorb and make use of nutrients.

However, each person in the advancing years of life displays a wide variety of individual changes. Although insufficient Vitamin E and a probable lack of oxygen in the bloodstream may be a major cause of aging, a person's specific needs should be determined under a doctor's care. Special conditions must always be considered when discussing general aging and general nutritional needs.

On the whole, however, the greatest influence of Vitamin E on the aging process takes place in earlier years. As we have noted, Vitamin E's most effective role is in the growth and middle years, which prepare us to meet the gradually declining metabolic processes of old age.

III To Be Young at Heart

The extremely painful chest pains that signal
an attack of angina pectoris have become a symptom of
our civilization. They are rightly feared, not only for the
extreme discomfort they cause, but because they may
foreshadow heart and artery disorders that can lead to
invalidism and even death. Vitamin E research provides
hope for a successful fight against the causes of angina.
Drs. Evan and Wilfrid Shute have found Vitamin E effective in improving the condition of eight out of ten patients
suffering from these attacks.

As Vitamin E influences the supply of oxygen within
the bloodstream, and as angina and related malfunctions
result from a lack in oxygen, the findings of the Shutes and
other medical authorities are of great importance. When
angina attacks persist, they may force a patient to give up
work, abandon all exertion, and eventually become a bed-
ridden invalid. If angina attacks continue over a longer
period, they may result in a serious coronary, either a
thrombosis (clot), a block, or an infarction (tissue deterioration because of insufficient blood supply).

The heart and artery diseases, known jointly as cardiovascular disorders, have greatly increased in number
during the past decades. Their victims are mostly men,

probably because male bodies require higher red blood cell values than women, while their bodies contain less. There are more deaths from heart disorders than from all other diseases combined. The problem is the same in the whole of Western society. Despite diligent research, the underlying causes of diseases of the heart and its vessels remain obscure, or a matter of dispute.

Vitamin E Therapy for Heart Disorders

Many factors are cited as contributing to heart disorders. Among them are such widely known conditions or habits as high cholesterol levels, overweight, lack of exercise, cigaret smoking, and such life crises as a man's worries about his job, friction with an employer and colleagues, or an abrasive home life. The list contains virtually all the hazards of modern civilization, including polluted air, lack of sleep, heavy coffee drinking, and a sedentary existence, to which TV watching has become a major contributor.

The widely cited causes of cardiovascular attacks are linked to imbalances in the diet. Too much cholesterol in the blood has been attributed to the high fat consumption of most Americans. Similarly, too many calories in our food and the excessive use of salt are blamed for some heart disorders. Therefore, the diet therapy adopted by most doctors for patients with heart disease focuses on the modification of these causes: fat, sodium, and calories. These food elements have been linked with such heart and arterial diseases as arteriosclerosis, congestive heart failure, hypertension, and actual heart attack.

In treating these major forms of heart disease, Vitamin E therapy has proved remarkably effective. Although cardiologists as a whole have held to their traditional ideas

16

and medication, refusing often even to test the effectiveness of Vitamin E for themselves, statistics recently released by Drs. E. Cheraskin and W. M. Ringsdorf, of the University of Alabama's Department of Oral Medicine, establish a definite correlation between Vitamin E intake and cardiovascular symptoms. Although the study group was limited to 299 persons, the evidence showed that a low Vitamin E intake was linked with a high incidence of heart symptoms and that an increase in this nutrient over a one-year period reduced the symptoms.

All but a few of the subjects were between the ages of thirty and sixty and consisted of dentists and their wives. Initially, each of them was given a dietary analysis. By having their subjects answer a "food frequency" questionnaire and submitting the results to computer analysis, Cheraskin and Ringsdorf were able to determine the average daily intakes of food and their specific nutritional value. The investigators confirmed that with advancing age there are progressively increasing symptoms of heart disease. However, they also determined that "Cardiovascular findings do indeed increase with age but only in those subjects consuming sub-optimal amounts of Vitamin E."

More startling was the conclusion the doctors drew from their findings when they observed the results of one year of Vitamin E therapy. They found that those who increased their Vitamin E intake experienced a "decrease in cardiovascular symptoms and signs," while those who "did not increase Vitamin E consumption did not improve with regard to the clinical picture." In advising its readers of the results of the Cheraskin-Ringsdorf experiments, the editors of the magazine *Prevention* remarked that "a daily intake of several hundred units (build up to this slowly, starting with 100) is the nearest you will ever come to insurance against coronary thrombosis." The reader should be cautioned, of course, that self-medication is always risky and that vitamin therapy should take place under the guidance of a qualified physician.

The work at the University of Alabama, as well as earlier experiments extending over a ten-year period, tends to confirm the general observations of Dr. Evan Shute on the manner in which Vitamin E acts on heart disease. He has noted that a patient who begins treatment on a full dose "will see no results for 5 to 10 days and often no really definite and measurable improvement for 3 to 4 weeks." If a patient starts from a small dose and increases it slowly, he will see "no results" until "after an effective dosage level" has had time to take full effect. But once improvement has started, Dr. Shute notes, it "continues for many months once the correct dosage has been reached and provided that there are no complicating factors." Such complications might be due to hypertension (high blood pressure) and hyperthyroidism (an overactive thyroid gland). He also cautions that too much Vitamin E can be prescribed for patients suffering from chronic rheumatic heart disease or from hypertension. No one affected by these illnesses should ever attempt self-medication.

Coronary Thrombosis

In the case of thrombosis, or a heart attack due to a blood clot, Vitamin E helps to dilate the capillaries and conserve oxygen. This reduces heart strain and keeps cellular tissues elastic. In addition to its ability to dissolve blood clots that have already formed, Vitamin E's anti-coagulant power also influences clotting time and thus tends to prevent improper clotting in the first place.

Unfortunately, coronary thrombosis is not only sudden

18

and often fatal, but even when the patient survives he is often crippled and may be expected to undergo another attack because, like a stroke, a thrombosis tends to recur. The reason why the most vital areas of the body, the heart and brain, are most often attacked is because there are fewer communicating branches between the arteries in those organs. As a consequence, in cases of coronary thrombosis it takes long for Vitamin E to reach individual cells in the brain and heart and perform its function adequately.

Both W. E. and E. V. Shute recommend that physicians prescribe a daily dosage of Vitamin E of at least 400 units for the normal person. For one suffering from a coronary artery insufficiency of any kind, a dosage of 800 to 1200 units of Vitamin E is suggested, depending on the needs and responses of the individual patients. The doctors expect improvement after six weeks of treatment, but suggest that the patient be kept on 800 units a day to assure the repair of any myocardial infarction (tissue damage to the heart) as well as to prevent clotting. Both doctors caution that if the prescribed dosage is not maintained indefinitely the patient may return to his previous condition within a week.

Neither doctor suggests that Vitamin E will be an effective control of every instance of angina, but they have personally treated more than thirty thousand patients in twenty-two years of practice and found that the vast majority of them were benefited. Only those patients whose conditions were so far advanced that they needed more blood and oxygen passing through their hearts than even Vitamin E could supply may be said not to have responded to some extent.

Hypertension

Tension and the modern life style have often been blamed for the tremendous increase in heart ailments. However, hypertension alone is not a disease. It is a symptom cluster that may be present in any number of cardio-vascular disorders. Although a common clinical problem, very little is known of its causes. "Hypertensive" is a general term used to cover a variety of heart diseases but is most often associated with high blood pressure. Some researchers have linked hypertension with sensitivity to high salt use, apart from other more general causes. A number of investigators have achieved clinical improvement of hypertensive patients through the use of a low salt diet. Special diet controls designed to establish a strict rice-fruit diet have been attempted, but the average patient finds it difficult to adhere to such a rigid regimen. Other clinicians have applied more liberal low sodium diets, keeping salt to 200 milligrams daily.

Regarding the use of Vitamin E in hypertensive cases, Dr. Wilfrid Shute has noted positive as well as negative results. He has carefully analyzed the special conditions and factors, and his report on the treatment of hypertensive cases contains cautionary observations addressed to his fellow physicians. Dr. Shute has noted that Vitamin E in "daily massive dosage led to rapid improvement in a good share of cases, with disappearance of the symptoms of failing heart action and even with a reduction of some blood pressures toward normal." In about one third of the cases, however, blood pressure "actually rose initially on such dosage, often to dangerous heights." The Shutes admit that they have been unable to sort out "distinguishing features in these hypertensive heart cases" which might

20

have made it possible to tell in advance "which patients would respond safely and in which cases the pressure would rise on such levels of medication."

It is clear from these findings that rare hypertensive heart cases do not initially benefit from Vitamin E therapy, and it is important to point this out to overenthusiastic supporters of this therapy who may come to regard it as a cure-all. Dr. Shute has pointed out that he and his brother have had more "failures" in the hypertensive group than in any other category of patients. And while he continues to believe that Vitamin E treatment should be considered in all hypertensive cases nevertheless, he is emphatic in warning against indiscriminate uses, stating: "In this type of case it is especially important that alpha-tocopherol should be prescribed by a physician with a thorough knowledge of its properties, lest real harm ensue." He regards it as "valuable prophylaxis against strokes."

Congenital Heart Disease

Unlike these cases involving hypertensive hearts, Vitamin E has shown itself to be uniquely valuable in the treatment of congenital heart disease. Although it can do little to improve the structure of the baby's heart, it can help the child to grow, prevent clots from forming (always a major problem in heart ailments), and reduce or relieve cyanosis (a condition in which the skin and membranes turn blue, as a result of improper oxygenation of the blood). Wilfrid Shute observes that Vitamin E is of "great value in those cases [of structural heart disease] which cannot be treated surgically. It is also the ideal treatment preoperatively and postoperatively for all those undergoing surgical repair."

For doctors who wish to run a test on the effectiveness

of Vitamin E, Dr. Shute recommends that the crucial cases they treat be those of mild to moderate cyanotic congenital heart disease or cases of fresh, acute rheumatic fever. Not infrequently patients with congenital heart disease also develop rheumatic heart disease after a period of rheumatic fever. "When this is suspected," he writes, "we immediately become more cautious in treatment and start such patients on smaller initial doses of the drug."

What About Cholesterol?

Hardening of the arteries—arteriosclerosis or atherosclerosis—is an underlying condition in much heart trouble, but its causes have not been satisfactorily defined. What actually happens is that deposits inside the artery walls narrow it, making blood flow erratic and eventually disrupting it. The search for the causes of these deposits has usually focused on the role that fatty substances play in the human metabolism. There are two reasons for this: (1) the artery-deposit formations are composed largely of cholesterol and other fatty materials, and (2) an elevated blood cholesterol level and an elevation of other blood fats is usually present. A number of researchers have shown a definite relationship between types of dietary fat and their effect on elevated blood fat levels. The substitution of foods high in polyunsaturated fatty acids for foods high in saturated fatty acids lessens the amount of cholesterol in the blood. However, what the significance of lowered cholesterol levels is in terms of the disease process is not clear. If the cholesterol level returns to normal, is further arteriosclerosis prevented? Is the progress of the disease reversed? No one knows, but doubts persist.

Hardening of the arteries is one of the most common and dangerous ailments of old age, although it is by no means limited to the elderly. Since the disease is usually well developed and has done its worst damage by the time it is detected, the low-cholesterol dietary regime is begun too late in many cases. The use of drugs to dilate, or widen, the arteries has had uncertain results, but a Russian team of doctors, headed by Dr. V. E. Anisimov, using 50 International Units of Vitamin E daily, obtained a definite improvement in the condition of patients suffering from arteriosclerosis and coronary sclerosis in conjunction with excessively rapid heart beat. Further evidence of the value of Vitamin E therapy in alleviating the symptoms of atherosclerosis comes from a group of Austrian doctors. They studied a group of nineteen women and sixteen men, whose ages ranged from fifty-four to eighty-two. These doctors administered 210 International Units of Vitamin E and 90,000 units of Vitamin A daily for a period of six months. Although this dosage, as Dr. Shute and others have discovered, is rarely sufficient in heart disease, the Austrian researchers noticed improvement after six weeks. Headaches, night pain, and insomnia, dizziness, a "ringing in the ears," and pain caused by walking—all symptoms of hardening of the arteries—were greatly relieved.

Seek a Vitamin Balance!

Just as these doctors prescribed Vitamin E in conjunction with another vitamin, so the reader should seek a vitamin balance and maintain it. A prime function of Vitamin E is to protect the other vitamins in the body, notably A and C since these vitamins oxidize easily.

Although tension and a high-cholesterol diet are popularly supposed to be most common causes of heart disease, there is a substantial body of evidence to indicate that this may not always be so.

23

This view was supported by the study of a group of forty-four Trappist monks, all past the age of forty, whose life of quiet meditation kept them free from daily tension and aggravation, and whose diet contained no animal foods except milk and small quantities of cheese. As might be expected their blood cholesterol level was lower than that of businessmen the same age. However, the study showed that in 59 percent of them there was some evidence of "retinal vascular disease," and that 48 percent of them suffered from high blood pressure.

Although no one would question the advisability of a relaxed mental attitude, a well-balanced diet, or plenty of exercise, it is a mistake to attribute heart disease to any one specific cause. Recent investigation has pretty well established that there is no single factor that causes heart disease in all people in all times and places. Yet it is well to bear in mind the suggestions of the American Heart Association: (1) Eat less animal or saturated fats; (2) Substitute unsaturated vegetable oils and other polyunsaturated fats for animal fats whenever possible; (3) Eat food low in cholesterol; (4) Avoid excessive weight and reduce the calory intake in your diet.

To these suggestions we must add the use of Vitamin E. Vitamin E acts on the heart and body cells like an oxygen tent. According to *Taber's Cyclopedic Medical Dictionary*, it "decreases oxygen requirements of heart muscles 50 per cent or more, increasing blood supply. It decreases excessive capillary permeability, or leakage; it reduces blood clot in thrombosis, or prevents its formation and softens scar tissue."

For those who have already had a heart attack, this knowledge of Vitamin E and its workings is of critical importance. However, it must be stressed again that the patient should not attempt to treat himself and that Vitamin E therapy is only effective when the patient has placed himself under a physician's care. Once therapy has begun, even someone highly vulnerable to heart attacks may take hope for a long and active life. No matter how scarred the heart muscle, no matter how thickened the arteries or how clotted the blood may be, Vitamin E provides a short-term and long-term prevention method by which the susceptibility to heart attacks is reduced.

IV   Toward a Vigorous Sex Life

Nutrition has been regarded as vital to healthy and long-lasting sexual happiness. But not always in the ways that men once thought. Madame Pompadour, for example, one of history's most celebrated courtesans, whose position at the court of Louis XV was unambiguous, believed that she could energize her amorous nature and sustain her physical charm with exotic diets. For breakfast she consumed truffle and celery soup, which she washed down with hot chocolate that had been laced with triple vanilla and ambergris. Unfortunately for the good lady, all she succeeded in doing was becoming overweight and dying at the even-then early age of forty.

However, at the other end of the scale, there is the Bulgarian peasant whose basic diet consists of two or three types of stews, and of whom roughly fifteen hundred out of every million live well past the age of ninety; in America only ninety people do so in the same sampling. Recently, one Bulgarian peasant who wished to sire another child was refused a marriage license because he gave his age as seventy. Investigation proved that he had falsified his age. He was actually ninety-three.

We often hear rumors of people who have lived to incredible old ages, sometimes past their two hundredth

26

year. They are rarely authenticated, however, and the record probably is held by Thomas Parr of London. Thomas only lived to be a hundred and fifty-two and he was buried in Westminster Abbey for that single, singular accomplishment. As a poor farmer he had no other claim to fame.

When he was presented in the court of King Charles I, the king inquired, "Parr, you have lived a great deal longer than do most. What else have you done that no other man has accomplished?" Parr replied that he had been displayed in the stocks as a public penance for promiscuous behavior. He had sired a child out of wedlock at the age of a hundred and five.

His young wife, who outlived him, was interviewed after his death and maintained that Parr had retained his full physical vigor until he was a hundred and thirty-two. After that he became blind and enfeebled, but not senile.

Vitamin E and Long Life

Vitamin E will probably not bring the reader the longevity of a Thomas Parr or substitute for the nutritious diets of the Bulgarian peasants, but it will enable him to realize a full and vigorous life span. The average American does not, at present, live longer than his ancestors, and according to the U.S. Public Health Service (1962) the national death rate has not improved in over a decade. As Herbert Bailey remarks the greater number of "senior citizens" today is due to less people dying from childhood diseases. "This fact does not mean, however, that the average man is living appreciably longer—it merely means that *more people* are living longer and, therefore, have a chance to exist until 70—or if their stamina is above average, they may live far beyond that."

Even though it has not increased to date, there is no reason why man's life expectancy should not. Dr. Paavo O. Airola expresses the view that Vitamin E plays a vital role in preventing aging, a view shared by numerous Russian scientists engaged in research on longevity. Dr. Olga Lepeshinskaya believes that the *normal* life span of the human being is potentially not less than a hundred and fifty years. And she reports, in *Life, Age and Longevity*, experiments with Vitamin E at the Institute of Biochemistry of the Russian Academy of Science have shown that "it has an enormously beneficial effect on the diseases of old age, specifically in combination with Vitamin A. The rejuvenating property of these vitamins has a direct effect on the sex glands. They also strengthen the ability of the tissues to absorb oxygen, restore impaired circulation in blood vessels, especially in the small capillaries, and help to restore the normal permeability of the blood vessels."

Dr. Edward L. Bortz, senior medical consultant, past president of the American Medical Society, and editor of the *Geriatric Digest*, shares the view that man's true life span may be a hundred and fifty years. Dr. Bortz distinguishes among chronological aging and biological aging, and psychological aging—all of which are necessary to our true understanding of what it means to "grow old." According to Dr. Bortz, our chronological age is marked by the calendar, which bears only a very rough correlation to our biological age at any time during our lives. Some people very advanced in years have body tissue and cells with the vitality of a thirty-year-old.

Obviously, it is our biological not our chronological age that matters. To keep our bodies in a youthful, healthful state, a well-balanced diet of natural foods, sufficient sleep, recreation, an enthusiasm for life and work, and a basic supplement of Vitamin E are necessary. With this program, we can at least expect that our psychological age will not be older than we actually are. A positive attitude toward life is essential, and with the proper care of our body's health, we can have it.

As we grow older, our psychological age depends more and more on the care we pay to our health. But it is also true that many of the ills of old age are psychosomatic in origin, caused by "old attitudes." A healthy mind in a healthy body; we cannot have one long without the other. "We should all have a justification for living," writes Dr. Bortz in *Creative Aging,* "that is of value both to ourselves and to society."

Vitamin E and Your Sex Life

Sexual activity is an essential part of human living. There is no valid biological reason for supposing it is the prerogative of any particular age group. Neither is there any definite number of times the sexual act may be performed and beyond which man's sexual nature will cease to function. Nor is the human need based entirely on the urge to procreate. It serves other, specifically human needs as well. As a means of self-realization, it is essential to the marriage relationship.

Vitamin E has been called "the reproductive vitamin," "anti-sterility vitamin," "the sex vitamin," and the "anti-miscarriage vitamin." However as Dr. E. Shute points out, this reputation for working miracles was acquired in early experiments with rats, not with humans. Although there is a mass of scientific evidence to show that deficiency in Vitamin E will cause heart failure, muscular distrophy, brain and neurological disorders, as well as reproductive failures, we should understand clearly what it can and cannot do.

In 1955, at the International Congress on Vitamin E

in Venice, P. L. Harris reported that when Vitamin E deficiency exists in rats, the testes degenerate and there is a decrease in both the sex hormones and in crucial gland activity. He also pointed out that the presence of Vitamin E protects the sex hormones from destruction by oxygen. Writing in *Vitamins,* Dr. Henry Borsook further distinguishes the powers of Vitamin E: "Severe vitamin E deficiency in men irreparably damages the tissues in the testes which produce sperm. No amount of vitamin E therapy can then repair the damage. Therefore such men become permanently sterile. . . . A woman who is severely deficient in vitamin E cannot carry a pregnancy through successfully. She has an early miscarriage. . . . In a woman, therefore, the harm done by a vitamin E deficiency is not permanent. She is not sterile."

In short, although Vitamin E can prevent sterility in laboratory animals, it cannot cure it. To call it the anti-sterility vitamin, therefore, is a mistake. It is even more misleading to think of it as the sex vitamin. It has no known direct effect on a man's sexual powers whatever; it is not an aphrodisiac. However, it does have an indirect effect on men's and women's ability to have successful intercourse, in that general health and well-being always have an effect on a person's sex life. Physicians have found that Vitamin E is able to revitalize the entire system, instilling it with new life and bringing about improvement in such illnesses of the later years as arthritis, heart troubles, diabetes, and failing eyesight.

The feeling of youth and well-being results from a process known as homeostasis. Carlson Wade describes this state in *The Rejuvenation Vitamin* as follows: "Your body and your mind live in a constant state of movement. Vitamins, minerals, enzymes and many other ingredients in the bloodstream both emphasize and control each other's functions; each body cell is kept in a state of dynamic equilibrium, endlessly changing each trillionth of a second to serve its own purposes and that of your body and mind as a whole." The contribution of Vitamin E to the body's youthful power of homeostasis is to rejuvenate body cells and so to "slow down" the aging process.

Vitamin E and Infertility

With the increased longevity and physical fitness, and remembering that Vitamin E cannot cure human sterility or enhance a man's sexual desires as such, does it really have any effect on the fertility of men and women?

The essential findings of the German physician R. Bayer, published in an Austrian medical journal, have been substantially corroborated by other researchers throughout the world, working with both animals and humans. Dr. Bayer reported of his studies with 100 married couples that when infertility first occurred, all of 144 conceptions had been lost prior to birth. Afterwards, the 100 couples achieved 79 pregnancies and only two of these women lost their babies. By using Vitamin E, Dr. Bayer was able to reduce the reproductive failure of his patients from 100 percent to 21 percent.

In cases of "secondary infertility," where there had previously been only 38 births out of 101 pregnancies, Dr. Bayer achieved the astonishing results of 41 pregnancies leading to 41 successful births—100 percent success. This was accomplished with his standard dosage of 100 milligrams of Vitamin E given daily to the husband for one month, and 200 milligrams given daily to the wife for three months prior to conception.

In order to prove that his results were the effect of Vitamin E intake and that alone, Dr. Bayer lowered the

Vitamin E intake of both groups to one third of its former potency. This produced an abrupt change. In the first group ("primary sterility") the loss of babies (which had been 100 percent prior to Vitamin E and 21 percent afterwards) became 33 percent because of the lower dosage. In the cases of "secondary infertility," the loss of babies was reduced from 61 percent (without Vitamin E) to 21 percent, instead of the 100 percent successful births with the original dosage. Husbands in the first group reported only a partial restoration of fertility; in the second group, the wife's fertility had only been partially established.

The work of Dr. Bayer and his associates suggests that not only is Vitamin E necessary for male and female fertility as well as the health of the offspring, but that the dosage must be of a definite amount in order to be therapeutic. Dr. Bayer's studies regarding the improvement in number and quality of sperm in the male, as a result of Vitamin E, have been corroborated throughout the world by other researchers.

The practice of Dr. Evan Shute, when he is consulted by couples that suffer from infertility or interrupted pregnancies, is to require an analysis of the male sperm, which may have been affected by a Vitamin E shortage. Dr. E. Lindner confirms the wisdom of this by noting an immediate increase in the male sperm count after treatment with Vitamin E. With a daily oral dosage of 150 to 200 milligrams of the vitamin, taken for a period of eight to forty weeks, normal semen levels were achieved by twenty patients, while another twenty-one showed definite signs of improvement. Of the twenty males who achieved a normal sperm count, seventeen were later able to impregnate their wives.

Dr. James W. Milten treated fifty patients twice daily with 30 milligrams of Vitamin E and twenty-three showed a marked increase in spermatozoa. In seventeen of these twenty-three men, there was also a marked increase in the volume of seminal fluid, as well as an improvement in the fluidity and strength of the spermatozoa and a decrease in abnormal forms. Dr. Shute notes that in twenty-seven cases of complete sterility or habitual miscarriages, ten conceptions took place (within a few weeks or months) following only three weeks of Vitamin E treatment.

We have concentrated in this chapter on the effect of Vitamin E in vitalizing the male partner, because countless experiments indicate that the male is responsible at least as often as the wife for an infertile marriage. He is very likely to be in part responsible for anomalies and habitual abortions in his wife. Vitamin E can thus be of great help to infertile marriages by improving the quality of the sperm count, thus increasing the number of healthy, active sperm.

Obviously, a man who is impotent, who cannot have successful sexual intercourse, is also functionally infertile. By helping to improve general physical and mental health, Vitamin E frequently can relieve impotence and thus remove this cause of infertility.

A word should be said here about the relationship of smoking to impotency. The man who suffers from impotence and who may also be taking sedatives, tranquillizers or alcohol, or smoking to excess, can conduct his own test by ceasing smoking for a trial period. Many men, upon giving up smoking, notice during the first few weeks a marked revival of their sexual potency.

Lung Disease

There is also a correlation between Vitamin E and lung disease. For this reason, the man who continues to smoke despite all medical advice should make certain of his Vitamin E intake each day. The key to Vitamin E's

33

role in preserving lung health was stated by Dr. Daniel B. Menzel and his associates at Battelle-Northwest, a research corporation. Vitamin E inhibits oxidation—that is, it prevents the chemical action of oxygen from combining with another substance, especially the pollutants nitrogen dioxide and ozone. Even when attacked by these pollutants, the unsaturated fatty acids in the lung tissue, that are essential to health, and especially Vitamin A, a highly unsaturated fat-soluble vitamin that oxidizes readily, are protected by the presence of Vitamin E.

Remember, age alone does not lessen a man's sexual activity, but poor health does. However, it would appear that maturer men stand in need of a greater Vitamin E intake in order to preserve the body's homeostasis and to slow down the aging process. No man for whom sexual activity remains important need fear its loss. Where his health remains good, the sex life usually continues unabated. Apart from its proven effectiveness in clinical cases involving the revitalization of the male sperm, the importance of Vitamin E in preserving the good health of every man cannot be stressed too strongly.

V   Vitamin E in Your Daily Diet

You have just come back from the health food store, and now a bottle of Vitamin E capsules stands right in front of you on the kitchen table. You pick it up and read the labels. One of them may state that the bottle contains Vitamin E "from d-Alpha-Tocopheryl Acetate," each capsule made up of 300 International Units. The bottle may contain 250 "Perles," which is their way of saying capsules.

You turn to the side of the label and read that the capsules are made "from vegetable oils." Under "Directions" you are told to take "As a dietary supplement providing Vitamin E, one perle daily." And finally the label states, "The minimum daily adult requirement of Vitamin E has not been established."

It is all very carefully worded, full of Latin words, and may use such terms as "biological assay" when telling you how the quantity of Vitamin E was measured. Sometimes the term "International Units," a worldwide measuring unit, is abbreviated as "I.U."

Where Does Vitamin E Come From?

Well, what does it all mean? The label, for all its cautious and elusive wording, is quite candid. The manufacturer suggests you take one capsule every day, and he tells you what's inside it; but he carefully refrains from stating whether you really need it, whether you need less or perhaps more than the 300 units. The packager can't prescribe the quantity of what he specifically calls a "dietary food supplement," because he does not know your body's condition and needs. He is not alone. Even your own doctor may not be able to say, off hand, whether or not you need the vitamin or how much you need daily— assuming he does agree with the basic idea that we need to add vitamins to our vitamin-depleted food intake. Of course, there are those who claim with a good deal of conviction that we get enough Vitamin E right in our normal diet, and that telling people to take vitamins is at best a mistake and at worst a racket.

As you look at those golden "perles," you wonder what they can do for you. How many should you take? Or does your daily food supply give you enough Vitamin E without any special effort. Some foods contain Vitamin E, but not much *alpha*-tocopherol, which is what matters most in heart and artery conditions, anemia and other physiological malfunctions. The various types of Vitamin E have been labeled after the first four letters of the Greek alphabet: alpha, beta, gamma, delta. Salad greens, for instance, contains gamma-tocopherol but no alpha to speak of.

Well, then, where's the real thing? In cereal grains. You get your important, alpha-type Vitamin E most directly if you bake your own bread from flour that hasn't been tampered with. This kind of homemade bread will spoil

36

easily, but you don't have the big food processor's problem of storing, shipping, and again storing bread, for days, weeks or months at a time. One reason the bread can be shipped and stored is that processors have learned to separate the spoilable wheat germ from the rest of the kernel. While this gives a big boost to the grain trade—China is able to get wheat all the way from Canada, for instance— it removes the alpha-tocopherol from the grain.

Maybe you don't have enough time to bake your own bread, or you can't get the unprocessed flour. Where else can you find Vitamin E in your daily food? Look for foods that contain oils extracted from cereal germs. You find them in vegetable margarines made from corn oil, soybean oil, wheat germ, or cottonseed oil. You also find them in the vegetable oils that you use in cooking or put on salads. The same goes for shortening made from vegetable oils. Look at your labels, most of them will be helpful, although some simply say the product contains "vegetable oil," but leave you to guess which cereal it comes from.

Some of the best things in life are neither free nor very stable. Vitamin E disappears the moment any of these oils turn rancid. Some ingredients that go into margarine, cooking oils, or shortening may play havoc with Vitamin E content. But there comes a point where you just can't worry about these details; your kitchen and body aren't chemical laboratories.

Still, you might as well know what foods are relatively high in Vitamin E, notably alpha-tocopherol, and which are not. The tables on pages 45-48 show this clearly. They first appeared in the *American Journal of Clinical Nutrition* of July 1965, where they formed part of a paper on "Alpha-Tocopherol Content of Foods." The authors are associated with the pharmaceutical firm of Hoffmann-LaRoche, Inc., of Nutley, New Jersey, which produces Vitamin E. The senior author, Dr. R. H. Bunnell, is biochemist and group leader in the company's Food and Agricultural Product Development Laboratory; two co-authors, J. Keating and A. Quaresimo, are analytical chemists in the same laboratory; a fourth author, G. K. Parman, was formerly assistant director in the firm's Technical Service Department. These researchers linked "the acceptance of Vitamin E as an essential nutrient in human nutrition" with the trend toward "polyunsaturated fatty acid" in our diets. The word "polyunsaturated" has become part of our vocabulary during the past ten years; it is a chemical term and usually refers to content of vegetable oils, as contrasted to animal fats. Vegetable margarine is polyunsaturated, as compared to lard. Anything that is in the polyunsaturated category has come to be considered a positive factor in modern nutrition.

Polyunsaturated Fats

How do Vitamin E and polyunsaturated fats act in relation to each other, now that we are eating so much more vegetable than animal fat? In 1946 the average person ate 10.5 pounds of butter each year. But by 1955 butter consumption was down to 9 pounds, and by 1963 to 6.8 pounds yearly. Just about the same has happened to lard. In 1946 the average person in the United States consumed 11.8 pounds of lard. This was down to 10.1 pounds in 1955 and 6.5 pounds in 1963. By now we may be down to 5 pounds or less per year, and our consumption of vegetable oils has increased in proportion.

It is an important switch. The New Jersey researchers compiled a table that showed how much more vegetable oils we now use in our margarine, in salad dressing, and in shortening. They broke this down into the main categories —soybean, cottonseed, peanut, and corn oil—but we will just give the totals, first in total pounds for the whole country, and then for the average person. In 1946 the country consumed only 474 million pounds of vegetable oils, and the average person ate 14.4 pounds of it each year. By 1955 consumption had more than doubled in the whole country, to 1,026 million, but this also had to do with the overall population increase; the average person consumed 17.7 pounds of vegetable oils per year. By 1963 overall United States figures came to 1,275 million, and the average person used 19 pounds per year. By now the quantity of vegetable oil each of us consumes on the average is probably far more than 20 pounds annually and may be closer to 25 pounds.

Loss of Vitamin E

On a good guess, we are putting four to five times more vegetable fats than animals fats into our food. In theory, this is fine for Vitamin E intake, because the oils taken from soybeans, cottonseed, and corn are high in Vitamin E, notably in alpha-tocopherol. The four researchers for the pharmaceutical company reaffirmed that "the most important sources of vitamin E in the diet are vegetable oils and foods containing significant amounts of vegetable oils or shortening." They reported, to any housewife's satisfaction, that "ordinary cooking processes used in preparing food for the table do not involve very large losses in tocopherol." However, a good deal of it gets lost "during the storage of foods which have been cooked in vegetable oils."

How did they find this out? They went to neighborhood grocery stores; they prepared fresh foods in their laboratory test kitchen, carefully following instructions on the packages; they kept control on storage and room temperatures; they chopped and mixed and blended. And to find out just how much tocopherol remained, to "assay" it (the word you read on the Vitamin E label), they used such new technological methods as gas-liquid chromatography.

Since many of our frozen foods are deep-fried in vegetable oil, one would think they might be high in Vitamin E. No, say Dr. Bunnell and his associates. They examined french fried potatoes, scallops, shrimp, and chicken cooked in vegetable oils or shortening, testing the assumption that "these foods should supply a significant amount of α-tocopherol in the diet." They discovered that "this is not so." And why? Because, while there is "little loss" during the actual deep-frying, there is "a great loss" in storage. This is even true when storage temperatures are low. Potato chips stored at room temperature lose a good deal of their Vitamin E, and chips as well as french fries lose it even when stored at extremely low temperatures.

The research team gives a chemical explanation for Vitamin E loss in storage, even at low temperatures. We needn't go into this in detail, except that they ascribe it to the destruction of tocopherol by hydroperoxides, even "during freezer storage despite good commercial packaging practices." They suggest that the vegetable oils should be strengthened with the addition of alpha-tocopherol acetate, a form of Vitamin E they describe as "stable to heat and oxidation."

Vitamin E in Your Foods

Now look at the tables these researchers have compiled, which put the results of their tests in graphic form. We have trimmed their original, scholarly tabulations down to what is essential to the consumer, eliminating the percentages of fat content and relations between tocopherol and fats. What you see, then, is the total tocopherol content in each food, given in percentages of milligrams, as well as the percentage of alpha-tocopherol.

The food chemists, interpreting the tables, wrote that fruits and vegetables obviously do not contribute significantly to the intake of Vitamin E in our diet. Canned vegetables are even less useful than fresh or frozen ones. Happily, home cooking of vegetables has only "a small destructive effect," while commercial processing and storage result in a "considerable loss." Meats, fish and poultry don't mean much to Vitamin E consumption, but of this group the fish are best and salmon steak best of all.

Naturally, desserts show a good deal of variety. Cookies and pies that utilize vegetable shortening "can be very good sources" of Vitamin E. Such snack foods as potato chips cooked in fresh vegetable oil can be "rich" in the vitamin. The sample menus the research chemists have analyzed show us how much or how little Vitamin E we get in our daily diet. These menus indicate an alpha-tocopherol intake ranging from 2.6 to 15.4 milligrams. That comes to an average daily consumption of 7.4 milligrams. This means that the "average" American diet contains actually only about half the daily Vitamin E intake that had been estimated earlier. This may be the result of changes in dietary habits or of differing research methods. At any rate, Dr. Bunnell and his associates think their findings point to a "relatively low" consumption of Vitamin E in at least "a portion of the population," depending, of course, on dietary habits.

Six Diet Rules

How do these findings affect your own diet and that of your family?

41

Here are the main points:

1. Avoid processed foods, and try to do your own deep-frying of such foods as shrimp, chicken, and potatoes.
2. Whenever possible, short-circuit the processing of food. So-called convenience foods may be convenient, but Vitamin E gets lost in storage.
3. Note that you do relatively well with a dish like broiled fresh beef liver but more than three times as well with oatmeal. Presumably, this is not the quick-cooking kind of oatmeal, although the researchers do not specify this.
4. Look for products based on cottonseed oils. In testing one margarine, Brand "B," as the researchers call it, a combination of cottonseed and soya oil showed 13 percent alpha-tocopherol. Mayonnaise and mustard also showed high percentages, but there is a limit to how much mayonnaise or mustard one can eat. (Cottonseed oil is a better source of Vitamin E than soybean oil.)
5. Whole wheat flour and unpolished rice, both of which have been emphasized by nutritionists for decades, retain much of their Vitamin E.
6. If you have not already done so, substitute vegetable fats for animal fats in your diet.

A Word of Caution

Your normal diet is, for the most part, not exclusively oriented toward Vitamin E. Our tables and summaries have nothing to do with other nutritional factors. Vegetable margarine may be just as high in calories, for instance, as butter. You may have to stay away from potato chips, for reasons having nothing to do with Vitamin E. And while there may be no harm in taking a capsule of Vitamin E per day (at that rate, it is presumably really just a dietary supplement and not a form of self-medication), you can't isolate it from the rest of your diet.

We are concentrating in this book on Vitamin E, and we know that we are tempting you into taking it on your own. We are convinced that a weak capsule a day is harmless and may well make you feel better. But when it comes to using it as a drug and not just to redress a diet imbalance, we are adamant in saying that you need a physician's guidance and prescription. Your own body is a special case, and you can't really deal with it exclusively from reading a book, even a completely frank book, like this one.

A good case can be made against taking Vitamin E alone. It seems to act best in concert with other nutritional elements. To keep a metabolic balance, Vitamin E might well be taken as part of a multivitamin tablet. The body tends to pick and choose from a minimum supply of vitamins. In the case of Vitamin E, it stores some of it in fatty tissues, while eliminating the rest. Vitamin C, on the other hand, is not stored at all and must be replenished in food or supplements constantly.

Good Nutrition Isn't Easy

You, as a reader interested in good nutrition, are torn between those who still insist that there is enough Vitamin E, or any other normally needed nutritional element in your food and those—like Dr. Bunnell and his associates—who seem to prove convincingly that food technology and buying habits are depriving us of more and more Vitamin E. But there are some obvious general conclusions. We do need Vitamin E. We have been getting less and less of it, beginning with processed bread and now reaching down to frozen deep-fried foods.

43

Therefore, aside from looking at your Vitamin E bottle and wondering whether you need the vitamin and how much you may need, keep these principles in mind. You cannot have ultra-convenience and good nutrition at the same time. If you must have bread that comes spoil-proof, sliced and handy on the supermarket shelf, then you cannot get maximum Vitamin E from your bread. If you prefer frozen deep-fried shrimp, rather than peeling and cooking the shrimp yourself in vegetable oil, you must allow for serious Vitamin E loss. These principles apply not only to Vitamin E, but to nutritional food values generally. The convenience foods not only cost more, but they also give you a package that is generally lower in the original nutritional values. Certainly it is preferable that you get your Vitamin E as directly as possible, right within your daily diet. The charts will tell you quickly where dietary weakness lies; it is up to you to reverse the process of Vitamin E deterioration in your own diet.

Vitamin E Content of Food

The following charts are based on more extended tabulations that accompanied the paper on "Alpha-Tocopherol Content of Food," by Bunnell, Keating, Quaresimo, and Parman, *American Journal of Clinical Nutrition* (Vol. 17, July 1965), and is reproduced here by permission.

Product	Total Tocopherol (mg. %)	Alpha–Tocopherol (mg. %)
Meats		
Bacon (fried)	0.59	0.53
Ham steak (fried)	0.52	0.28
Pork sausage (fried)	0.32	0.16
Liverwurst	0.69	0.35
Bologna	0.49	0.06
Salami	0.68	0.11
Ground beef (pan fried)	0.63	0.37
Fresh beef liver (broiled)	1.62	0.63
Fresh veal cutlet (pan fried)	0.24	0.05
T bone beef steak (broiled)	0.55	0.13
Lamb chops (broiled)	0.32	0.16
Pork chops (pan fried)	0.60	0.16
Fish		
Fillet of haddock (broiled)	1.20	0.60
Salmon steak (broiled)	1.81	1.35
Deep-fried frozen shrimp		
Oven heated	6.6	0.6
Not heated	5.9	1.9
Deep-fried frozen scallops		
Oven heated	6.2	0.60
Not heated	3.9	0.71
Poultry		
Chicken breast (broiled)	0.58	0.37
Frozen fried chicken Brand "A"		
Oven heated	0.32	0.04

Product	Total Tocopherol (mg. %)	Alpha–Tocopherol (mg. %)
Poultry (continued)		
Brand "A-1"*		
Oven heated	1.39	0.38
Not heated	1.43	0.40
Brand "B"		
Oven heated	1.10	0.16
Not heated	0.80	0.10
Vegetables		
Raw potato	0.085	0.053
Baked potato	0.055	0.027
Boiled potato	0.061	0.043
Frozen french fried potatoes		
Brand "A"		
Oven heated	0.36	0.12
Not heated	0.64	0.15
Brand "B"		
Oven heated	1.59	0.43
Not heated	1.22	0.41
Fresh yellow onion	0.34	0.22
Frozen french fried onion rings		
Brand "A"		
Oven heated	6.2	0.72
Not heated	5.2	0.60
Brand "B"		
Oven heated	6.4	0.65
Not heated	5.5	0.52
Baked beans, Boston style	1.16	0.14
Fresh peas	1.73	0.55
Canned green peas	0.04	0.02
Frozen green peas		
Cooked	0.65	0.25
Uncooked	0.64	0.22
Canned green beans	0.05	0.03
Frozen cut green beans		
Cooked	0.25	0.11
Uncooked	0.24	0.09

*Same as "A" but bought at a different store.

Product	Total Tocopherol (mg. %)	Alpha–Tocopherol (mg. %)
Vegetables (continued)		
Canned leaf spinach	0.06	0.02
Canned kernel corn	0.09	0.05
Frozen kernel corn		
Cooked	0.48	0.19
Uncooked	0.49	0.19
Celery	0.57	0.38
Carrots	0.21	0.11
Lettuce	0.17	0.061
Fresh tomatoes	0.85	0.40
Dry navy beans	1.68	0.47
Cooked white rice	0.27	0.18
Fruits and Fruit Juices		
Fresh strawberries	0.29	0.13
Frozen sliced strawberries	0.40	0.21
Fresh banana	0.42	0.22
Fresh cantaloupe melon	0.31	0.14
Fresh apple	0.51	0.31
Canned tomato juice	0.71	0.22
Canned grapefruit juice	0.18	0.04
Fresh orange juice	0.20	0.04
Breads		
White bread	0.23	0.10
Whole wheat bread	2.2	0.45
Cereals		
Oatmeal	3.23	2.27
Corn flakes	0.43	0.12
Dry processed rice cereal	0.28	0.04
Dry oat cereal	1.53	0.60
Yellow corn meal	3.43	0.64
Hominy grits	1.17	0.31
Processed wheat and barley cereal	2.45	0.61

Product	Total Tocopherol (mg. %)	Alpha–Tocopherol (mg. %)
Desserts		
Chocolate ice cream		
Brand "A"	1.02	0.36
Brand "B"	1.10	0.37
Vanilla ice cream	0.39	0.06
Fresh baked apple pie	15.7	2.50
Fresh baked blueberry pie	17.7	3.12
Fresh pound cake	7.4	1.1
Chocolate cupcake	2.0	0.14
Milk chocolate bar	4.2	1.1
Peanut butter/oatmeal cookie	7.67	6.0
Shortbread cookie	1.33	0.46
Wafer type cookie	1.43	0.53
Chocolate/cream cookie	2.81	1.29
Miscellaneous		
Mustard	4.15	1.75
Whole milk	0.093	0.036
Butter	1.0	1.0
Egg	1.43	0.46
Corn oil margarine, brand "A"	46.7	13.2
Soya and cottonseed oils margarine, brand "B"	59.5	13.0
Cocktail peanuts	11.2	6.7
Dry roasted peanuts	11.7	7.7
Instant coffee	0.48	nil
Cottonseed oil mayonnaise, brand "A"	9.0	6.0
Mayonnaise, brand "B"	50.0	24.3
Polyunsaturated mayonnaise, brand "C"	42.0	8.6
Potato chips	11.4	6.4
Pretzel sticks	0.77	0.15
Club cracker	1.17	0.80

Alpha-Tocopherol
Content of Typical Menus

Breakfast—1

	Serving (g.)	Alpha–Tocopherol (mg.)
½ medium cantaloupe	150	0.21
1 cup cooked yellow corn meal	28*	0.18
1 slice white bread	23	0.02
1 pat butter	10	0.10
3 strips bacon	23	0.12
1 egg	54	0.25
coffee and sugar		nil
4 oz milk for cereal and coffee	120	0.04
Total		0.92

Breakfast—2

	Serving (g.)	Alpha–Tocopherol (mg.)
½ cup tomato juice	100	0.22
1 cup cooked hominy grits	40*	0.12
2 slices white bread	46	0.04
2 pats margarine, brand "A"	20	2.62
1 egg	54	0.25
coffee and sugar		nil
Total		3.25

Breakfast—3

	Serving (g.)	Alpha–Tocopherol (mg.)
3¼ oz orange juice	100	0.04
1 oz corn flakes	28	0.03
2 slices white bread	46	0.04
2 pats margarine, brand "B"	20	2.60
coffee and sugar		nil
4 oz milk for cereal and coffee	120	0.04
Total		2.75

*dry weight

Alpha-Tocopherol
Content of Typical Menus

Breakfast—4

	Serving (g.)	Alpha–Tocopherol (mg.)
3¼ oz grapefruit juice	100	0.04
2 slices white bread	46	0.04
2 pats butter	20	0.20
2 sausages	40	0.06
1 egg	54	0.25
coffee and sugar		nil
Total		0.59

Breakfast—5

	Serving (g.)	Alpha–Tocopherol (mg.)
3¼ oz orange juice	100	0.04
1 cup dry processed rice cereal	28	0.01
2 slices white bread	46	0.04
2 pats butter	20	0.20
2 slices ham	60	0.17
1 egg	54	0.25
tea and sugar		nil
4 oz milk for cereal and tea	120	0.04
Total		0.75

Breakfast—6

	Serving (g.)	Alpha–Tocopherol (mg.)
½ cup tomato juice	100	0.22
¾ cup cooked processed wheat and barley cereal	30*	0.18
2 slices whole wheat bread	46	0.20
2 pats margarine, brand "A"	20	2.62
2 slices ham	60	0.17
1 egg	54	0.25
coffee and sugar		nil
4 oz milk for cereal and coffee	120	0.04
Total		3.68

*dry weight

Alpha-Tocopherol
Content of Typical Menus

Breakfast—7

	Serving (g.)	Alpha–Tocopherol (mg.)
3¼ oz grapefruit juice	100	0.04
1⅛ cup dry oat cereal	28	0.17
1 slice white bread	23	0.02
1 pat margarine, brand "B"	10	1.30
3 strips bacon	23	0.12
1 egg	54	0.25
coffee and sugar		nil
4 oz milk for cereal and coffee	120	0.04
Total		1.94

Breakfast—8*

	Serving (g.)	Alpha–Tocopherol (mg.)
½ medium cantaloupe	150	0.21
2 slices whole wheat bread	46	0.20
2 pats butter	20	0.20
2 links sausage	40	0.06
2 eggs	108	0.50
coffee and sugar		nil
Total		1.17

Luncheon—1

	Serving (g.)	Alpha–Tocopherol (mg.)
3 slices liverwurst	90	0.33
2 slices whole wheat bread	46	0.20
7 leaves lettuce	50	0.03
1 medium tomato	150	0.60
1 tablespoon mayonnaise, brand "B"	13	3.16
1 slice pound cake	30	0.33
1/6 qt chocolate ice cream	95	0.34
6 oz milk	183	0.07
Total		5.06

*Average Alpha-Tocopherol content of eight breakfast menus = 1.88 mg.

Alpha-Tocopherol
Content of Typical Menus

Luncheon—2

	Serving (g.)	Alpha–Tocopherol (mg.)
1 large hamburger	82	0.30
10 pcs french fried potatoes, brand "A"	50	0.06
½ cup canned peas	80	0.02
1 slice blueberry pie	160	4.99
coffee		nil
Total		5.37

Luncheon—3

	Serving (g.)	Alpha–Tocopherol (mg.)
3 slices bologna	90	0.06
2 slices white bread	46	0.04
7 leaves lettuce	50	0.03
mustard	10	0.18
1/6 qt vanilla ice cream	95	0.06
6 oz milk	183	0.07
Total		0.44

Luncheon—4

	Serving (g.)	Alpha–Tocopherol (mg.)
4-6 deep-fried shrimp	50	0.30
1 tablespoon mayonnaise, brand "A"	13	0.78
10 pcs french fried potatoes, brand "B"	50	0.22
½ cup frozen peas	80	0.20
3 shortbread cookies	75	0.36
1 chocolate bar	50	0.55
coffee		nil
Total		2.41

Alpha-Tocopherol
Content of Typical Menus

Luncheon—5

	Serving (g.)	Alpha–Tocopherol (mg.)
2 slices whole wheat bread	46	0.20
3 strips bacon	23	0.12
7 leaves lettuce	50	0.03
1 medium tomato	150	0.60
1 tablespoon mayonnaise, brand "C"	13	1.02
10 potato chips	20	1.28
1 medium banana	150	0.33
3 wafer type cookies	75	0.39
6 oz milk	183	0.07
Total		4.04

Luncheon—6

	Serving (g.)	Alpha–Tocopherol (mg.)
1 pc veal cutlet	92	0.05
½ cup navy beans	100	0.47
3 x 5″ stalk celery	50	0.19
10 pcs french fried potatoes, brand "A"	50	0.06
1 slice pound cake	30	0.33
15-17 roasted peanuts	15	1.16
6 oz milk	183	0.07
Total		2.33

Luncheon—7

	Serving (g.)	Alpha–Tocopherol (mg.)
2 slices white bread	46	0.04
3 slices salami	90	0.09
mustard	10	0.18
7 leaves lettuce	50	0.03
7 pretzel sticks	10	0.02
½ cup frozen strawberries	100	0.21
1/6 qt vanilla ice cream	95	0.06
6 oz milk	183	0.07
Total		0.70

Alpha-Tocopherol
Content of Typical Menus

*Luncheon—8**

	Serving (g.)	Alpha–Tocopherol (mg.)
1 fillet of haddock	105	0.63
1 cup white rice	168	0.30
½ cup canned spinach	90	0.02
½ cup frozen corn	83	0.16
1 slice pound cake	30	0.33
6 oz milk	183	0.07
1 medium fresh apple	150	0.46
Total		1.97

Dinner—1

	Serving (g.)	Alpha–Tocopherol (mg.)
½ medium cantaloupe melon	150	0.21
2 slices beef liver	74	0.47
½ cup canned kernel corn	83	0.04
10 pcs french fried potatoes, brand "B"	50	0.22
1 cup canned green beans	125	0.04
1 medium fresh banana	150	0.33
2 chocolate/cream cookies	23	0.30
coffee		nil
Total		1.61

Dinner—2

	Serving (g.)	Alpha–Tocopherol (mg.)
3¼ oz grapefruit juice	100	0.04
2 pork chops	140	0.24
½ cup carrots	75	0.08
1 cup white rice	168	0.30
½ cup canned spinach	90	0.02
1 medium fresh apple	150	0.46
1 peanut butter/oatmeal cookie	75	1.50
coffee		nil
Total		2.64

*Average Alpha-Tocopherol content of eight luncheon menus = 2.79 mg.

Alpha-Tocopherol
Content of Typical Menus

Dinner—3

	Serving (g.)	Alpha-Tocopherol (mg.)
½ cup tomato juice	100	0.22
T bone steak	120	0.16
french fried onion rings, brand "A"	50	0.36
½ cup baked beans	130	0.18
½ cup fresh peas	80	0.44
½ cup frozen strawberries	100	0.21
1/6 qt vanilla ice cream	95	0.06
tea		nil
Total		1.63

Dinner—4

	Serving (g.)	Alpha-Tocopherol (mg.)
Salmon steak	100	1.35
1 cup white rice	168	0.30
½ cup frozen kernel corn	83	0.16
½ cup canned peas	80	0.02
2 chocolate cupcakes	120	0.16
coffee		nil
Total		1.99

Dinner—5

	Serving (g.)	Alpha-Tocopherol (mg.)
¼ broiled chicken	85	0.31
1 cup white rice	168	0.30
½ cup fresh peas	80	0.44
1 slice white bread	23	0.02
1 pat margarine, brand "A"	10	1.31
1 slice apple pie	160	4.00
coffee		nil
Total		6.38

Alpha-Tocopherol
Content of Typical Menus

Dinner—6

	Serving (g.)	Alpha–Tocopherol (mg.)
¼ frozen fried chicken, brand "B"	85	0.14
10 pcs french fried potatoes, brand "A"	50	0.06
1 cup frozen green beans	125	0.14
7 leaves lettuce	50	0.03
1 medium tomato	150	0.60
1 tablespoon mayonnaise, brand "A"	13	0.78
1 slice white bread	23	0.02
1 pat butter	10	0.10
1 slice pound cake	30	0.33
coffee		nil
Total		2.20

Dinner—7

	Serving (g.)	Alpha–Tocopherol (mg.)
5-6 deep fat fried scallops	145	0.87
1 tablespoon mayonnaise, brand "C"	13	1.02
10 pcs french fried potatoes, brand "B"	50	0.22
french fried onions, brand "B"	50	0.33
½ cup frozen peas	80	0.20
1 slice whole wheat bread	23	0.10
1 pat butter	10	0.10
2 chocolate cupcakes	120	0.16
coffee		nil
Total		3.00

Dinner—8*

	Serving (g.)	Alpha–Tocopherol (mg.)
2 lamb chops	70	0.12
½ cup baked beans	130	0.18
½ cup frozen kernel corn	83	0.16
½ cup carrots	75	0.08
3 x 5" stalk celery	50	0.19
1 slice whole wheat bread	23	0.10
1 pat margarine, brand "B"	10	1.30
1/6 qt vanilla ice cream	95	0.06
2 chocolate/cream cookies	35	0.30
tea		nil
Total		2.49

*Average Alpha-Tocopherol content of eight dinner menus = 2.74 mg.

VI Evan and Wilfrid Shute: Pioneer Brothers

The city of London, Ontario, is situated just above the Canadian border with the United States. It lies within the so-called Golden Triangle of its three large neighbors, Toronto, Detroit, and the Niagara area. It is a proudly Canadian town, but in a larger sense it is North American, a union of industrial and cultural interests that link the United States and Canada. It is appropriate that the two embattled pioneers of Vitamin E, Dr. Evan V. Shute and his brother, Dr. Wilfrid E. Shute, should have brought controversial medical prominence to this crossroads of U.S.-Canadian life. Evan Shute has said bitterly, "How lucky we have been to live in Canada! I know how long we would have lasted in territory controlled by the American Medical Association. How many valuable ideas in medicine must have died aborning because its authorities made the going too heavy and young men have simply given up."

The Shutes, rugged men in their sixties, are stubborn and vocal. They feel certain that their own treatment of nearly forty thousand patients has given ample proof that their claims for Vitamin E are fully justified; that researchers in Latin America, Europe and Asia have duplicated and bolstered their own results; and that mankind is much the poorer and sicker for not using the vitamin that is needed as a dietary supplement or in larger, controlled doses for specific therapy.

In his busy office at 10 Grand Avenue in London, Evan Shute says calmly, "I think I haven't even been tough enough in print; I keep on being polite, and pulling my punches." The Shutes' mood is one of civilized anger. Vitamin E, they believe, has suffered from the same foolish scientific lag that delayed the acceptance of such vital substances as penicillin, insulin, and Vitamin C. Penicillin developed from the unlikely origin of a mold grown from the air that was injected into a patient's muscle to cure bacterial infections in the lungs, tonsils, or abdomen. Evan Shute recalls that the basic concept of penicillin "sounded so fantastic that it took fourteen years and the Second World War for medical men to give it a trial!"

The Shutes also remind us that the distinguished Canadian Sir Frederick Grant Banting—who practiced medicine in London and set up the Banting Research Institute in Toronto—made medical history with insulin, the substance that controls diabetes. "Imagine," writes Evan Shute in *The Heart and Vitamin E,* "removing the pancreas of a slaughtered animal, then extracting a fluid which could be injected under the skin of humans to help the body use any sugar not properly handled by the patient's own pancreas." In his introduction to his book, Evan Shute notes that that, precisely, "is what Banting did and what he announced to the medical world."

One more example, and one well known even to high school students, is scurvy, the debilitating disease of sailors whose diet was limited to foods that could be salted and dried for long journeys. This illness was traced to lack of citrus fruit, and limes were added to the diet of British sailors (thus giving us the slang epithet "limey"). That was back in the sixteenth century. Only in 1933 was Vitamin C, or ascorbic acid, fully identified in citrus fruit and pine needles. Is it any wonder that the Shutes are irritated at the prospect of such a delay in the medical acceptance of Vitamin E?

Reluctant Medical Acceptance

But are they right? Can all those prestigious medical societies be wrong? Not only has the American Medical Association ignored or resisted the Shutes' claims for Vitamin E, the doctors have had similar trouble in Canada itself, although it has not interfered with their own treatments or research. When their work had been under way for less than a decade, the Canadian magazine *Macleans* (June 15, 1953) made a survey of popular and professional reactions to their work. The author of the article, Eric Hutton, noted that while the claims of the Shutes appeared to be detailed and well documented, "many other Canadian doctors, eminently qualified and eminently reputable, either discount the Shutes' claims for Vitamin E entirely or maintain that the claims have not yet been scientifically proved." Today, some twenty years later, the words "not yet" are still being used by many in the medical profession, although hundreds of new entries are added to the extensive bibliographies of scholarly works on Vitamin E.

The Ontario College of Physicians and Surgeons has maintained that Vitamin E "has no place in the treatment of cardiovascular disease"; while the Canadian Medical Association, taking a more neutral stand, said that it did "not endorse or condemn the use of this substance in the hands of the medical profession" and expressed the polite hope that it will "find its true place in the realm of thera-peutic agents when physicians of the world have made a careful appraisal in their own practice and based on their own observation."

The Shutes, frankly, would like to see general recogni-tion of Vitamin E's qualities in their own lifetimes. They are not patient men, and they have grown more impatient with the medical establishment as evidence of Vitamin E's manifold healing qualities accumulates.

There is a psychological difference between, for in-stance, the acceptance of Vitamin C as a cure for scurvy and related disorders and the acceptance of a vitamin with such varied uses as Vitamin E. Medical professionals as well as laymen almost automatically resist anything that sounds like a cure-all. This argument, too, annoys the Shutes, who point to cortisone, a twentieth-century wonder drug that is used routinely in the treatment of such diverse disorders as arthritis, allergies, and gout.

The impatience that powers the Shutes' drive for recog-nition of Vitamin E runs counter to the self-consciously deliberate, ritualistic research approach in medicine and other scientific disciplines. The establishment resists short cuts. It wants to see the channels of academic bureaucracy respected. It reacts negatively to any research stardom, a tendency that was apparent even when Dr. Jonas Salk developed the vaccine that virtually wiped out infantile paralysis. The Shutes' irascible nature may be partly responsible for the resistance they have encountered. Doc-tors, who have to play God to their patients most of the day, are not conditioned to be called to task for alleged ignorance or negligence. Evan Shute recognizes that when he says that "perhaps the discovery was never to blame—only the discoverers." Still, if the Shutes hadn't been stub-born and persistant, Vitamin E would probably never have received the worldwide attention that it has. It is in the nature of messianic discoverers, ever since it was claimed that the earth is round, to antagonize the established order.

A Family of Physicians

Vitamin E is in many respects a Shute family enterprise. Any good public relations adviser might have told them not to call their research body The Shute Institute for Clinical Laboratory Medicine but to leave their family name out of it. But the story of their lives and work does have family roots. In fact, their own mother, then seventy-two years old and invalided by a severe heart condition, was her son's second patient. She told Eric Hutton, the author of the *Macleans* article, that the results of the treatment were "like a miracle," and that she improved so much that "I could do things I hadn't done for years, even tend the furnace." Evan Shute, proud that they could give their mother many additional years of useful life, adds wistfully that if this had been the only result "of all we have gone through, then it has been fully worth it."

The Shutes are a family of physicians. The father of Wilfrid and Evan, Dr. R. James Shute of Windsor, Ontario, was a general practitioner. He experimented with certain thyroid extracts that had some relation to Vitamin E. Later his son Evan, an obstetrician and gynecologist, working with the aid of a scholarship from the Banting Institute, found that thyroid extract and Vitamin E both acted as "antagonists" to the female hormone estrogen, which meant that its level in the bloodstream could be controlled. Evan Shute encountered a number of cases of apparently preventable miscarriages among his patients. His interest was shared by Dr. Earl Watson of Victoria Hospital in London, Ontario. Both physicians were stimulated by an article in the British medical journal *The*

Lancet, which seemed to offer a promising direction. The journal reported on the use of Vitamin E by the Danish veterinarian Philip Vogt-Miller to prevent repeated miscarriages, so-called habitual abortion. The implication was that there was something basically wrong with the internal balance of a woman who had multiple miscarriages; studies at the Universities of California and Arkansas had drawn similar conclusions a decade earlier.

Evan Shute was successful in research and therapy dealing with threatened miscarriages, using Vitamin E. It was during this period of pioneer experimentation in 1937 that he used Vitamin E first in a patient suffering from severe angina pectoris. The Shutes recall that they were lucky in that this particular patient was able to respond to Vitamin E in low quantities. Also, as it was then only available as a wheat germ oil product, it was helpful that the patient could swallow the oily substance without becoming nauseated.

A dramatic case came their way in 1948, when the Shutes and a student, the late Dr. Floyd Skelton, were looking for a patient suffering from purpura, bleeding under or within the skin. They found such a patient in the care of Dr. Arthur Vogelsang. The man was not regarded as fit for an operation because of a severe heart condition. With Dr. Vogelsang's cooperation, Skelton and Evan Shute started Vitamin E therapy.

Dr. Vogelsang went to see this patient a week later at the hospital and was chagrined when he found that his bed was empty. As the case had been serious, the physician upbraided the nurse for not having notified him of the patient's death. The nurse, however, simply pointed to the other end of the hospital floor, where the patient was busy helping the nurses in their chores. Evan Shute recalls that obviously "the patient's heart condition had been helped even more than his purpura."

It is a valid caution, at this point, to note that Dr. Vogelsang, who carried on Vitamin E research for an extended period, said that he had become a "conservative advocate" of Vitamin E and believed "that many cases of certain types of heart and arterial disorders will respond to proper treatment within Vitamin E, often in combination with conventional agents." Dr. Vogelsang also stated: "But this treatment is a form of chemotherapy—the use of a chemical to obtain a therapeutic effect. There is no logical reason to believe that heart or arterial diseases are caused by a dietary deficiency of Vitamin E, and therefore I prefer to call the stuff by its chemical name, alpha-tocopherol. It can be dangerous in inexperienced hands, and therefore I deplore publicity which might tempt laymen to start self-treatment with Vitamin E."

The Case of the Family Barber

The Shutes' careers are filled with similar case histories. The early ones have a fine parochial feeling, the more recent ones are more cosmopolitan. But there is no substitute for the hometown touch of the case of their barber, Roy Bicknell. He was a member of the Shutes' church, the Reorganized Church of Jesus Christ of the Latter Day Saints (this is *not* the better known Mormon Church of Utah, but traces itself to an original group that remained in the east, while the others moved westward). As Evan Shute told Hutton, the author of the *Macleans* article, Bicknell had nothing to lose from trying Vitamin E, as his heart doctor had stopped treating him and simply told him to take some morphine tablets if the pain became unbearable.

"His legs were swollen," Shute recalled, and "his distress was so great he could scarcely tolerate the weight of his pajama top on his chest. He could not lie down but sat up night after night gasping for breath. Twenty-three days after I started him on Vitamin E he was back playing in the London Little Theater orchestra, working in his shop, and going fishing."

Medical Iconoclasts

Wilfrid Shute, the cardiologist, reported by 1970 "The number of patients whose treatment I have supervised personally or through other doctors working at The Shute Institute now exceeds 30,000." Wilfrid, the younger of the two brothers, is as outspoken as Evan. And while Evan also has the distinction of being an ordained minister in his church, Wilfrid is renowned as Canada's top judge at dog shows and a leading breeder of Doberman Pinschers. He is athletic, fond of sports and the outdoors, and showed these preferences when he married Dot Prior, a swimming champion who represented Canada at two Olympic games. Their daughter is also an expert swimmer. All three of them use Vitamin E in their daily diets.

There are no ifs and buts in Dr. Wilfrid Shute's appraisal of the status of Vitamin E today. "By now it is possible to say with complete assurance," he states, "that alpha-tocopherol is a thoroughly tried and tested therapeutic agent, unusually successful in its results, and with its effects so well defined that it can be used with precision by any competent physician." He maintains that doctors can deal with acute kidney inflammation, acute rheumatic fever, and acute thrombophlebitis (blood clots) in 48 to 96 hours. He insists that such cases, when treated as soon as diagnosis is complete, "will be, by all criteria, laboratory and clinical, completely cured in two to four days!"

64

It is not surprising that the medical profession, used to a more cautious vocabulary, seeks to ignore or discredit such claims. The younger Dr. Shute feels that doctors should include Vitamin E in their therapy as a routine element. "Such a potent drug," he urges, "if it had no other value than in the treatment of such cases, is an absolute necessity in the armamentarium of every doctor, whatever his specialty or type of practice." The doctor, he says, must suit the dosage to his patient's requirements. Except for inorganic iron, mineral oil, and female sex hormone, Vitamin E can be mixed with other treatments. Specifically, it can be used side by side with nitroglycerine, the anti-hypertensive drugs, and with diuretics, which reduce the water held within the body and thus counteract swellings.

What makes the Shutes such iconoclasts to the medical profession is their criticism of some apparently tried-and-true concepts in dealing with heart disease. They have a sure knack, as the saying goes in England, for "putting the cat among the pigeons." After many years of casting about for basic causes of heart conditions, many medical authorities have come to believe that cholesterol may play an important part in creating deposits that narrow artery walls. They have also shown a tendency to blame the tempo of modern living for causing tension and stress, which in turn contribute to the vastly increased number of deaths from heart attacks. Dr. Wilfrid Shute, writing in *Vitamin E for Ailing and Healthy Hearts,* challenged these assumptions: "If our ancestors could live on isolated farms threatened by Indian raids and not get coronaries, stress can hardly be bad for the heart." He believes that "before the turn of the century there was more stress involved in caring for larger families on lower earnings; an employee was unprotected before the whims of his boss and knew that if he lost a job it might take months, years or forever to find another." Actually, Dr. Shute states, there are very few stresses today that were not present in what he calls "pre-thrombotic times."

Vitamin E and Heart Disease

Shoveling snow after a blizzard may be bad for you, and so may be an excess consumption of animal fats, but maybe you are vulnerable to these and other factors—stresses, dietary errors—because Vitamin E has been progressively removed from our foods since the days of our pioneer ancestors, or at least since the turn of the century. The intake of animal fats has gone down, but it is not clear that this has reduced the incidence of heart disease. Wilfrid Shute notes that "there is much evidence to suggest that there is no relationship between dietary fat and coronary artery disease, although the therapy still has its adherents." Cutting down on animal fats in the diet is probably beneficial in general. It is generally accepted that it is better for one's heart and general health to be fairly lean, but controversy still rages throughout the medical world about the effect of cholesterol on the heart and the arteries. Dr. Shute obviously feels that it is unwise to emphasize this one dietary factor while ignoring the need for Vitamin E. He cites a case that illustrates this point dramatically.

One of Dr. Shute's neighbors, an apparently healthy and athletic man, had been playing hockey with his son during the 1967 Christmas holidays. While they were playing, the man was struck by severe chest pains. Alarmed, he stopped and had his son help him into the car. While driving home he started to vomit and barely managed to get to his house. Dr. Shute found him on the upper floor of his home; he had not managed to reach his bed. He was taken to the hospital, where Shute gave him sedation and

66

medication to dilate the arteries, but he remained in pain for nearly twenty-four hours. Dr. Shute also administered 1,600 units of Vitamin E and this regimen was continued daily. The electrocardiogram pointed to a clot in the left artery of the heart.

This patient "had for years carefully watched his weight and diet, retaining a trim figure free of any hint of obesity." The man exercised daily and took a two-to-three-mile walk nightly, had never smoked, did not drink, and had even avoided "late hours and carousing" at convention hotels. He was bitter that, after all this, he should be felled by a heart attack.

Wilfrid Shute reported the incident in his book in particular detail, because it showed that a "clean life" is not enough to guard against heart attacks, but that Vitamin E is essential. Shute told his patient that all these preventive measures were not enough, as long as "the bloodstream is deficient in the nutritional content that should naturally be there." In other words, all the clean living was in vain, because the body under stress just did not have the needed weapon, Vitamin E, with which to defend itself against a heart attack.

VII "But Will It Erase My Wrinkles?"

While doing research for this book, members of our editorial team could not help but express their enthusiasm to others, often in dramatic terms. One of us, finding himself seated next to his charming middle-aged hostess at the dinner table, discovered that he was dominating the conversation with quotations from medical journals, tales of remarkable cures, and other bits of colorful vitamin lore. He was brought up short by his hostess's sudden question, "But will it erase my wrinkles?"

Our researcher, himself safely middle-aged and long trained to turn such cosmetic questions into compliments, decided to forego an easy conversational exit such as "Twenty years from now, when that question may really arise, nutrition will have made this problem nonexistent." Instead, he gave his hostess a quick and self-consciously appraising look and decided to be honest with her and with himself. So he said, "I don't know, but I'll try to find out."

Can Vitamin E really influence such effects of aging as the crinkles and folds that mark the human skin? Wrinkles, after all, start with the newborn baby whose body is covered with a wet and blotchy skin that hardly seems to fit at all. Right from the start there are wrinkles where they are obviously needed: on the palms of the baby's hands, the soles of the feet, inside the elbow. In later years, as tissues lose their youthful flexibility, wrinkles turn up in other places. Gaining weight, thereby stretching the skin, then losing weight and leaving the skin with less surface to cover, is common. Our habit of seeking a suntan, which means drying the skin and actually hastening the aging process, also contributes to wrinkling, as do characteristic facial expressions, frowns, laughter, everything that reveals emotions or moods on our faces.

External Use of Vitamin E

Should our hostess have worried about her wrinkles at all? In this day of the cosmetic facelift, of almost exaggerated emphasis on youth, a natural way of slowing down such telltale signs of aging as wrinkling is no longer simple vanity; it reflects a desire to keep external appearance in line with an inner agelessness, which is entirely desirable and attractive.

The claims for Vitamin E are so numerous and, let's face it, often so fantastic-sounding, that we hesitate to be dogmatic about the vitamin's cosmetic potential. But the evidence that points toward such a potential is too fascinating to be ignored. Dr. Wilfrid Shute tells of the experience he and his brother had of applying the vitamin as an ointment directly to the skin. This method has been effective in dealing with burns, ranging from "the small domestic burn, due to contact with a heated iron or a stove burner or scalding steam and water, to the most severe third degree burn." Dr. Shute noted that such treatment may seem "far afield from the heart," with which Vitamin E is most closely identified. What happened in cases of burns is particularly significant, because it made skin grafting unnecessary and obviously aided the body's normal healing functions in a manner that cannot be explained easily.

It is startling to discover that a substance that acts in many subtle ways *inside* the body can be applied effectively from the *outside* as well. Most people tend to doubt and suspect such multiple function. But Dr. Shute quite rightly noted that Vitamin E is not alone in this dazzling versatility. He cites the example of ACTH and cortisone, which are "used in so many apparently diverse and unrelated areas of medicine." The mere fact that Vitamin E is effective when taken orally does not mean it cannot also work when applied externally to the human skin.

One indication of the possible impact of orally-taken Vitamin E on rejuvenation of the skin comes from the Shutes' observation that "patients all notice that their fingernails and toenails grow more rapidly, as does hair." There is, of course, a direct link between the growth of nails and hair and their dermatological base, the skin itself. Vitamin E also tends to step up glandular activity, including perspiration, which adds moisture to the skin. There is, in fact, a body of data that tends to support the notion that Vitamin E can have a positive impact on the human skin, certainly where the healing process and basic vigor are concerned.

The Skin: The Body's Largest Organ

When our researcher's hostess raised the simple question about her wrinkles, she actually asked a whole series of questions to which few definite answers are known. The skin is the largest organ of the human body, a complex chemical unit that covers us from head to toe and is made up of several layers. When we talk about wrinkles, we are just thinking of the most external covering, the outer layer known by its Latin name, *stratum corneum*.

While cosmetics, the scented cleansers, moisteners, and cover-ups produced by the beauty industry, are designed to be applied to this outer skin, we must never forget that our skin is an area of two-way flow. It signals heat and cold, moisture and dryness, the impressions conveyed by touch—with all their emotional aspects—and keeps the body in balance by its network of pores through the elimination of water by perspiration. What we see as the outer skin is actually in a constant state of peeling. The skin is in perpetual transition, as cells are pushed outward from the lower strata and eventually dry out and fall off.

In other words, skin is not just an outward armor that might be made to look better by polishing and lubricating. You cannot fix it like the finish of a car, with a good washing and waxing job. It dries out as a result of being exposed to the sun's rays; it tans as pigmentation changes and it becomes smooth when oiled; its pores open to warm water and close to cold water. But at the same time other processes are being carried out underneath the outer layers.

We now come to the blood vessels that are just below the most important growing area; you need no Latin to understand the meaning of its name, *stratum germinativum*. Here the cells of the skin germinate, are formed and then move outward in a continuous living, growing stream. This stratum of self-renewal is characteristic of the whole body, but outwardly most noticeable in that body's largest organ, the skin. The perpetual turnover of skin cells is made possible by the fertilizing action that extends from the blood vessels through a network of tiny extensions, the papillae, into the outer levels of the skin.

It is this dynamic aspect of the skin, we eventually told

71

our hostess, that explains how Vitamin E can help her avoid wrinkles. One way is by application of the vitamin as an ointment, from the outside. The other way, of course, is the one with which we are now familiar, the use of Vitamin E as a nutritional supplement that acts most dramatically in keeping the body's blood supply in optimum condition.

The knowledge of what makes the skin behave, what makes it ill or well, is still quite limited. Anyone who has consulted a dermatologist about a routine complaint such as itching or eczema may well have experienced a whole series of trial-and-error treatments, ranging from radiation to a wide variety of salves and liquids. Mature medical men are ready to admit that their knowledge is still limited, and dermatologists are among those most eagerly awaiting results of ongoing research.

Meanwhile, we have to live with whatever knowledge does exist, and when it comes to outward signs of aging— folds and furrows in the human skin—we might as well use all available means at our command. It is probably too much to ask that even Vitamin E, versatile as it is, actually "erase" wrinkles. That would mean reversing a complex process that has been under way since early childhood. But would it not be enough if the consistent nutritional use of Vitamin E, combined with use of the vitamin as an ointment, could actually *delay* these unsightly outward signs of aging?

The Skin and Emotions

Wrinkles are not just indentations in the skin that come, soon or late, deep or shallow, all by themselves. Once we understand their relationship to the delicate chemical balance within the bloodstream, to the ever-changing content or flow of blood, then we see the skin as protector and signal for the whole body. The skin is enormously responsive to the seesawing of emotions. Blushing, the chill of fear, the little hairs standing on end with excitement—all such responses show the relationship between emotion and skin action. The rushing of blood to the surface of the skin or the feeling that your blood is "running cold" are physiological expressions of emotional ups and downs. Although many rashes and other chronic or temporary skin disorders may be caused by allergic reactions or viral or bacterial infection, it is also possible that many skin disorders have an emotional basis and are in fact physiological expressions of anxiety, frustration, or anger.

Vitamin E can assist the body in combatting what we might call emotional aging. If we consider the most fully established function of the vitamin, its contribution to the quality and flow of blood within the body, we can find a direct link to two vital aspects of human life: (1) actual physical and mental disintegration, and (2) the fear of old age and death. It is important to realize that even the most superficial masking of the aging process can provide at least a brief emotional uplift. If Vitamin E can help delay or even reverse such outward aging symptoms as wrinkles, then it can also have an emotional impact. It can give a woman—or man—a new lease on life by preventing the outward appearance from signaling the growing-old process. Skillfully applied cosmetics can achieve this, at least temporarily, but Vitamin E may well create a condition that actually delays the aging process, so that the outward appearance becomes a direct reflection of the underlying health and continuing youthfulness.

There appear to be numerous indirect links between the bodily functions of Vitamin E and a person's mental well-being. We must emphasize that Vitamin E acts in concert with many other factors, and it may not be able to override stronger elements. Glandular functions, which have an important impact on such basic conditions as the fatty secretions of the skin, may contribute to dry and wrinkled skin. Or environmental factors, ranging from an abrasive family life to anxiety-inducing urban living, may bring about the stresses that hasten aging. Vitamin treatment usually has little or no effect on these factors.

Vitamin E and Skin Health

Our hostess asked, perhaps a little mischievously "But will it erase my wrinkles?" Although we assume her question was both frivolous and serious, we feel it is important that women understand that wrinkles are not necessarily a bad thing. A certain amount of lines and creases reflects character, experience, humor, and warmth. An adult face that looks like a store-window dummy's is not beautiful. Thus we are not really determined to stamp out wrinkles completely. But we are seriously concerned with the biochemical conditions of which they are a symptom, and we can see that a relatively youthful face may help to bring about an emotional equilibrium that springs from the self-confidence a good-looking person enjoys. Depending on one's body chemistry, life style, and heredity Vitamin E can play many roles in contributing to this equilibrium. Beyond the answer to a half-mischievous question lies the ultimate truth that the human skin is both a guardian and a barometer of human health.

It is probably fair to extend the comments on the use of Vitamin E for superficial wounds to speculation on its possible impact on the aging process as it affects the skin. Dr. Wilfrid Shute noted in *Vitamin E for Ailing and Healthy Hearts* that it is probably a good idea to take it by mouth while also applying it to the body externally. He put it this way: "The oral administration of alpha-tocopherol should be begun simultaneously with the topical ointment, since, while either alone may be effective, one complements the other." He also reported, in this context, that Vitamin E in ointment form "apparently penetrated intact skin" and is of "real value in relieving itching of skin." The Shutes have applied the vitamin in vanishing cream, not for cosmetic uses but in the treatment of discomfort caused by a varicose vein, and to treat charges in the external genitalia especially.

The clinical evidence, then, points toward the fact that Vitamin E should be regarded as potentially helpful in counteracting prematuring aging of the skin. Treatment of such serious skin difficulties as burns suggests that it may be useful to apply it in ointment form. At the same time, by acting through the bloodstream, Vitamin E affects cell formation and helps to replace the cells on the outer layer of the skin. This two-way approach gives the body the benefit of the vitamin's healing-lubricating qualities in ointment form, while providing it simultaneously with the nourishment that acts as an anti-aging factor throughout the whole body.

Have we answered the question of whether Vitamin E can "erase" wrinkles? To put it quite simply: it may not be able to erase them retroactively, but there is a good chance that Vitamin E can help keep them from getting more numerous, or from showing up too early, in the first place.

VIII Needs During Pregnancy

We saw in Chapter V the effects of Vitamin E on male infertility; now we will look at the relationship of Vitamin E to the fertility and pregnancy of the female partner. Naturally, since the concerns of the two partners cannot be separated, there will be some overlapping between the two chapters.

We have already noted the improvement of the sperm count in the male as the result of increased Vitamin E intake. In order to insure the health of their offspring, the woman, guided by her gynecologist, should take an intensive course of Vitamin E therapy for at least three months before attempting conception. In this way she will be better assured of carrying her child for the full nine months and avoiding many of the troubles that beset women during pregnancy. For the purposes of his general health and to avoid the heart attacks that are most prevalent among the male population, the father should continue to take Vitamin E, even though his role in the production of a healthy child is now completed.

"The Pill" and Vitamin E

Since many of the women wishing to conceive will have just stopped taking birth control pills, let us consider the relationship between the pill and Vitamin E. There has been a great deal of medical literature about the increased dangers of cancer, thrombophlebitis, and other illnesses in women taking contraceptive pills, and it seems fairly well established that such dangers exist. Dr. Wilfrid Shute notes that "just as every patient whose doctor has put him on a polyunsaturated fat diet needs increased vitamin E, so does the woman who takes the pill." He observes that by adding the vitamin "she reduces virtually to zero the danger of thrombophlebitic complications." He answers the question of how large a daily "preventive quota" of the vitamin there should be, stating that such a figure has never been computed "with any degree of accuracy or with anything like a full knowledge of the nature of Vitamin E deficiency disease." His "educated guess" comes to 200 international units daily "for the adult in normal good health."

Under normal conditions, Vitamin E reduces the blood's formation of thrombin, the clotting agent that tends to reduce the likelihood of thrombosis. However, with an intake of estrogen, one of the hormones in contraceptive pills, a woman may neutralize the effect of Vitamin E. It appears also that the vitamin tends to regulate the formation of fibrin, the blood protein that normally causes blood to clot. With the use of estrogen, the collection of fibrin becomes greater and so do the chances of thromboembolism.

Writing in *The Rejuvenation Vitamin* of the other risks the pill incurs, Carlson Wade notes that "without vitamin

E, cellular wastes and blood lipids [fats] may join with oxygen to form" compounds that "may bring about premature aging, not to mention reproductive and fertility disorders." He adds that "liver ailments, digestive disorders, chronic tiredness and impaired mental ability" may also result. Wade states: "More severe side effects from this hormonal tampering include excessively high blood pressure, jaundice, an abnormal increase in blood glucose that may be similar to diabetes and even strokes."

For the woman who has stopped using the pill or other birth control devices and wants to become pregnant, Dr. Edmond J. Farris, of the Wistar Institute of the University of Pennsylvania, suggests the following procedure in the *American Journal of Obstetrics and Gynecology:*

1. For the three months of Vitamin E therapy, the woman should count her menstrual cycle. Beginning with the end of one cycle, count to the beginning of the next. Add the figures for each of the three months and divide by six. The resulting number will give you the number of days from the end of your cycle until the midcycle day.

2. Two days before that midcycle day, engage in coitus once a day for three days (in other words, including the midcycle day). Five days prior to the first coitus in this series, the male and female should engage in coitus, and then abstain until this three-day cycle begins. This practice assures the greatest activity and strength of the sperm.

3. This practice should be continued for four months. If the desired conception does not take place, the entire schedule should be moved *back* one day. If after another four months, conception has still not occurred, put the schedule *ahead two days*.

4. Throughout the three-day cycle, since she may very well not always find herself in the mood, it is not

expected that the female will reach her climax; but it is necessary that she should experience enough excitement to have normal glandular secretions.

Naturally, consultation with a gynecologist should precede any such regimen, and it should not be applied as self-medication.

Nutrition in Pregnancy

Once impregnation has been achieved, it is essential that proper nutrition be continued, since the development of the infant is directly related to the diet of the mother. However, experience has shown that greatly varying diets have sustained individual mothers through successful pregnancies, and medical literature reports conflicting and often controversial observations concerning the expectant mother's nutritional requirements. Each woman must follow her own needs and the advice of her physician.

This is especially necessary because for centuries all over the world a great deal of folklore has surrounded pregnancies. Many women still continue to follow traditional practices and diets that have little foundation in fact. Even a great deal of clinical advice is still based on supposition. It was not until the 1920s that medical literature began to outgrow dogmatic beliefs and to reflect scientific experiments and careful observation. Research first indicated that pregnant women should eat a varied diet and avoid excessive weight gain. Soon thereafter, the concept developed that a child is "nutritionally nine months" old at birth. In 1943, the National Research Council first published its recommendations for dietary allowances. These allowances have undergone continuous revisions, reflecting the continuing uncertainty in the area of prenatal feeding.

This controversy surrounding the diet of the pregnant woman, which began in the 1920s and 1930s, continued to grow in the 1940s and 1950s. During this period many researchers brought forth what appeared to be conflicting evidence concerning the influence of the maternal diet on the health of the child.

Despite these fluctuations of medical opinion, the value of Vitamin E for the expectant mother is no longer seriously challenged. Indeed, the relationship between Vitamin E and the reproductive process has long been known among primitive peoples. During the time of the Old Testament, for instance, Jewish custom prescribed a pregnancy diet high in Vitamins E, A, and D, consisting of wheat, barley, parched corn, beans, lentils, olives, butter, honey, lamb, the cheese of kine, fatted fowl, and oxen, and fruits of the field.

Controlling Miscarriages

The value of Vitamin E for the pregnant woman was carefully explored in the early 1930s. And many studies have been undertaken since then. In a recent study three groups of women were kept under close observation. As reported by Henry Borsook, in *Vitamins,* the first group, thirty-five women who had previously had two or more spontaneous miscarriages, were each given one-half teaspoonful of wheat-germ oil daily. Twenty-five of them carried their pregnancy through successfully. Another eleven women, each of whom had experienced one miscarriage, were given the same dosage; nine completed their pregnancy successfully. A group of nineteen women faced miscarriages during the first three months of pregnancy. Their dose of wheat-germ oil was increased to one tablespoonful daily, and thirteen of them achieved successful pregnancy.

Exactly how does Vitamin E work to reduce the probability of habitual abortion, or miscarriage? To answer this question we should refresh our minds on what occurs during a miscarriage. In a normal pregnancy, the fertilized ovum attaches itself to the uterine wall, from which it draws nourishment. A thick tissue or placenta develops, and from it extends the umbilical cord to the navel of the fetus. Inside the cord there is a vein and an artery for carrying blood to and from the fetus and the placenta. The placenta itself rests in a pool of blood which it has created by eating away the uterine wall.

In a successful pregnancy there is a balance between the eroding ferments of the placenta and a counteracting substance, which it also produces and which keeps it from eating through the uterine wall. In other words, it eats into the wall deeply enough to gain an adequate supply of blood for the fetus, but not so deeply as to perforate the wall. Although most early miscarriages represent Nature's way of ridding the body of a defective conception—and thus are a good thing—some miscarriages occur when the balance of nature is destroyed as a result of the placenta producing too much of the counteracting substance and never developing a firm attachment to the uterine wall.

The effect of Vitamin E is to reestablish Nature's balance by neutralizing the counteracting substance and permitting the digestive elements of the placenta to eat their way into the uterine wall deeply enough so that the placenta will not separate prematurely.

Dr. J. Edward Morison feels that Vitamin E helps not only prevent miscarriages, but also stillbirths, toxemia, and a rapid destruction of the red cells known as hemolytic anemia. We have already noted the anti-oxidant function

81

of Vitamin E for the reproductive system and its conservation of body oxygen so that blood and tissue cells are kept at their fullest health. In connection with pregnancies, it should be noted that an absence of life-giving oxygen in the placenta for even a short period can cause brain damage in the child.

Since the health of the fetus depends so greatly on the mother's blood, an unimpaired circulatory system is essential for a healthy successful pregnancy. Vitamin E helps to keep the veins in the body from becoming clogged and also to improve the blood flow. To this extent the danger of phlebitis is lessened and therefore the mother-to-be is not so apt to be afflicted by the swollen tissues, high blood pressure, and overall appearance of having aged, which normally occur after phlebitis.

Vitamin E and Premature Birth

In his book *The Heart and Vitamin E,* Dr. Evan Shute states that Vitamin E "seems able to rescue a considerable proportion of women who threaten to terminate their pregnancies too soon, the percentage rising as the period of gestation advances. Thus in the last two months of pregnancy over 70 per cent of precarious cases may be rescued, and a corresponding group of women may remain pregnant even after early rupture of their membranes and appreciable loss of the watery fluid which normally cushions the infant in the womb."

The role of Vitamin E in the prevention of premature births is not really different from that of preventing miscarriages. Although many American women still believe that even when a woman suffers during pregnancy, Nature takes care of her child by supplying it with nourishment, albeit at her expense, the facts are otherwise. A study made at the Boston Lying-In Hospital by Drs. Burke, Beal, Kirkwood, and Stuart indicated that when the mother's nutrition is inadequate during pregnancy the fetus suffered more than the mother. In this survey of 216 women, all stillborn and premature, all "functionally immature," and indeed all infants who died within a few days after birth, with one exception, as well as all of those suffering from obvious congenital defects, had mothers whose diets during pregnancy were inadequate. Conversely, mothers whose nutritional intake was good produced infants in fine physical condition.

For several years, a number of tests involving premature infants have been conducted by Dr. F. Gerloczy of the University Medical School, Budapest. He found that disorders ranging from scleroderma (a water swelling, usually following an infection and frequently fatal) to abnormally slow growth were most common where there was a Vitamin E inadequacy and that the seriousness of the illness was in direct proportion to the vitamin deficiency. In 320 cases the fatality rate of premature children with scleroderma was 75 percent. With Vitamin E therapy the rate of death dropped to 27 percent.

Vitamin E and Infant Disease

Researchers throughout the world have found evidence supporting Dr. Gerloczy's findings and noted that among the most frequent afflictions of infants, especially premature ones there was a definite lack of Vitamin E. In most cases, when the infants were put on Vitamin E therapy, the conditions cleared up. A joint medical team from Mount Sinai Hospital and Johns Hopkins School of Medicine found that infant diseases of the gall bladder and pancreas were helped significantly by

Vitamin E therapy. At the University of Freiburg, Germany, Dr. R. Beckman discovered that Vitamin E produces similarly helpful results in infants suffering from diseases of the liver. He also suggested that 300 milligrams of Vitamin E given to the mother before the onset of delivery reduces the possibility of brain hemorrhage in the infant. All of these doctors recommend supplemental intakes of Vitamin E for infants, especially those who are not breast-fed.

Similar results have been found by nutritionists and physicians among premature babies deficient in Vitamin E. If one assumes that premature births are at least partly due to a vitamin deficiency in the pregnant mother, the sequence of events becomes clear. The baby, in its prenatal state, has only limited access to oxygen. But at the moment of birth this balance changes drastically: oxygen begins to enter the lungs and bloodstream as direct breathing begins. The impact of relatively large amounts of oxygen can cause a rapid breakdown of essential fatty acids. The early administration of Vitamin E counteracts this condition, reducing the destructive impact of oxygen on fatty acids and tends to establish a biochemical balance.

According to an account in *Pediatrics* (1954), Dr. W. C. Owens, Johns Hopkins Medical School, gave 150 milligrams of Vitamin E to twenty-three premature babies; these did not become blind, while one-fifth of another group of premature babies, who did not receive the special vitamin treatment, lost their sight. When vitamin treatment began at the age of six weeks, the infants tended to become nearsighted. The precise impact of Vitamin E on the infants' sight may have to be determined by additional research under still more controlled experimental conditions. Overoxygenation of premature babies is regarded as a major cause of eye damage, as the babies frequently have to be put into oxygen tanks.

Vitamin E and Birth Defects

We have already seen the importance of Vitamin E for the proper functioning of the heart in adults; the administering of Vitamin E in proper dosage to the newborn infant is not less important. Approximately twenty-five thousand children (.3–.5 percent of all live births) are born each year with congenital heart disease. This figure does not include babies born with structural defects of the heart that occur along with other malformations of the body. But regarding these structurally defective children, or "anomalies" as they are known technically, and their tendency to recur in certain families, Dr. Evan Shute observes: "It has been estimated, for example, that if one child in a family is thus defective at birth, the chances of another brother or sister being structurally defective are increased by 7 times, or to about 1 in 7— from the 'norm' we have found (for our particular locality) of one in 45 births. Great success has been reported where the sire of such families has been given alpha tocopherol *before all subsequent conceptions.*" Obviously, the would-be parent who is prone to produce anomalies should prepare for conception with an intensive Vitamin E therapy course.

That improper nutrition may be one of the causes of these malformations appears very likely from the data collected by Professor Oscar Erf concerning domestic animals, as well as from an article by F. P. Mall which appeared in the *American Journal of Anatomy*. Dr. Mall states that out of nearly 100,000 pregnancies that he studied in England "80,572 were normal births, 11,765 abortions of normal embryos and early monsters, and 615 monsters born at term." Most impressive in the work of these two researchers is the close similarity between human and animal anomalies such as the clubfoot, the cleft palate, jaw malformations, and dental malocclusion.

Danger of Toxemia

Perhaps the greatest danger to the mother and infant resulting from impaired blood flow (uterine ischemia) is toxemia. This is perhaps the most soundly based assumption of the causes of toxemia, although Eastman and Helman have studied in depth some thirteen theories of its cause. One of the most serious and common ills of pregnancy, toxemia is often referred to as "the enigma of obstetrics" and the "disease of theories." Its reality remains quite grim. Several researchers have presented clinical and laboratory evidence that toxemia is a disease of malnutrition which can damage the liver and affect its metabolic activities. Toxemia is often found in women whose pregnancy diets are inadequate in vitamins.

Toxemia usually occurs in the third trimester, the three months just preceding birth. Among its clinical manifestations are swelling (edema), hypertension, the presence of albumen in the urine (albuminuria), and, in severe cases, convulsions and coma. Occurring usually after the onset of the twenty-fourth week, toxemia may bring about such symptoms as convulsions and coma. A more common and closely related variety of toxemia is chronic hypertensive (vascular) disease, which may exist in some patients before pregnancy or may occur before the twenty-fourth week and persist until after childbirth.

Specific treatment of either of these forms of toxemia varies according to the symptoms and needs of the individual patient, but optimum nutrition is a fundamental aspect of therapy. The first type of toxemia comes suddenly and the patient rapidly goes into convulsions. The more common hypertensive form is less dangerous and rarely results in death, but the illness tends to kill the unborn child, usually by separation of the afterbirth. It is this more common form of toxemia which seems to be prevented or eased by Vitamin E. "Alpha-tocopherol tends to anchor the afterbirth in the second and common type of toxemia, perhaps providing better local circulation in this organ, which is the basic circulatory and nutritive organ of the yet-unborn infant. It is widely believed that the afterbirth is the source of the toxins or such other agents which damage mother and child in these 'toxic' states. Presumably an afterbirth kept from degenerating by an improved circulation is less apt to release such noxious agents. Increased oxygenation, too, must play a role, for the unborn child lives at levels of oxygen intake on which no adult could survive. These can readily drop to concentrations too low even for the child." As we have seen, the oxidizing effects of Vitamin E make it a sound precaution against such a misfortune.

Although there is much dispute within the medical profession regarding the origin and treatment of toxemia, the value of Vitamin E is evident and the need for further research more evident still. Six to 7 percent of all pregnancies present cases of toxemia. It accounts for the majority of all maternal deaths (about 1,000 in the U.S. annually), and for the majority of all the deaths of newborn infants (roughly 30,000 stillbirths and neonatal deaths per year). With proper attention to sound nutrition and an adequate intake of Vitamin E and other vitamins, which should be part of good prenatal care, many of these deaths could be avoided. The good nutrition that a woman brings to her pregnancy, and maintains throughout it, provides her with the best chances for adapting to the physical stresses of gestation. Her fitness for and during pregnancy is a direct result of her past nutrition.

Preparing for Pregnancy

Writing in the *Ohio State Medical Journal,* Dr. James B. Patterson strongly urged the use of Vitamin E in wheat-germ oil for a healthy pregnancy. "Any patient who threatens to abort is a deserving candidate for some form of therapy. Obviously, prophylaxis [prevention] if available would be better management. Such an approach has been made possible by the use of a concentrate of wheat germ oil."

While statistics on the application of Vitamin E treatment are sometimes difficult to evaluate, there does seem a strong tendency toward an improvement in the "quality" of the baby born to parents receiving Vitamin E treatment. In hundreds of such treatment cases, as far as available records show, there is no case of a defective or mentally retarded child. This points toward a healthier sperm, as well as toward generally better conception and pregnancy conditions from which the developing fetus is able to benefit.

In this chapter we have considered the effects of Vitamin E during and before pregnancy. But how can Vitamin E contribute to the continuing health of mother and child after birth, and, most especially, what is its contribution to their health during the nursing stage? The next chapter considers the nutritional importance of Vitamin E for the newborn child and the mother.

IX Feeding the Infant and Child

A 1942 survey of 514 mothers in Philadelphia showed that only 43 percent of these women had good diets with adequate vitamin supplements and that only 48 percent had normal deliveries. The other women experienced major complications during pregnancy and were not able to achieve spontaneous delivery. In addition, they produced children with low birth weights and they had difficulty establishing adequate milk supply in the hospital. The mother's diet is an important factor in successful childbirth and in the postpartum period. Although it is difficult to establish any correlations between specific nutritional deficiencies and particular difficulties in delivering a child, it seems certain that women who experienced nausea and morning sickness during early pregnancy and numbness in the legs, fatigue, and muscle spasms in the later months—common ills for mothers-to-be with the generally deficient American diet—were receiving too little Vitamin B_1 or thiamin, and Vitamin E, as well as suffering from a generally inadequate vitamin intake.

Vitamin E and Diseases of the Newborn

When the mother has not had a sufficient amount of Vitamin E during pregnancy, the infant may suffer from jaundice as a result of the red cells in his body breaking down upon exposure to oxygen. As soon as Vitamin E is added to the infant's diet, the destruction of these cells ceases and the jaundice disappears.

There is also a possible relationship between Vitamin E and the possibility of brain damage to the newborn child, as well as muscular dystrophy and other afflictions of the central nervous system. Dr. Lyon B. Stream has noted: "Lack of oxygen for even short periods could produce brain damage to the fetus. General anesthesia for childbirth should be reduced to a minimum for the prevention of brain damage to both mother and child."

For the infant whose mother has not had the proper consumption of Vitamin E, a delay of only a few minutes before he begins to breathe may be sufficient to injure his brain permanently because he has not been able to store up a sufficient oxygen reserve. As Carlson Wade observes "For an infant having to rely for a whole minute on the residual supply of oxygen it has received from its mother, an ample supply of Vitamin E with the consequent conservation of oxygen in its natural state may be a matter of life and death."

Still another infant illness caused by a Vitamin E deficiency is anemia. Dr. M. W. Dick-Bushnell, of the University of Wyoming, investigating why anemia often occurs in bottle-fed babies and continues for several months after birth, discovered a considerable lack of Vitamin E in infant formulas and baby foods. The breast-fed baby does not suffer from breaking down of the blood cells when the mother has had sufficient intake of Vitamin E during pregnancy and shortly before delivery.

Vitamins During Breast Feeding

The physical strain of lactation (breast feeding) is even greater than that of pregnancy. The nursing mother therefore requires more dietary additions, especially Vitamin E, than does the pregnant woman. The lactating mother herself may require an increased quantity of Vitamin C, although the dosage her doctor recommended during pregnancy may suffer, since milk contains little Vitamin C. Increases over the mother's predelivery intake are suggested, however, in the B-complex vitamins, riboflavin and niacin (about a one-third increase over the quantities taken during pregnancy), in Vitamin A and its necessary correlate, Vitamin E (2,000 international units more). Since these vitamins are important coenzyme factors in cell respiration, glucose oxidation, and energy metabolism, the need for increased quantities of them increases with the caloric intake. However, for maximum efficiency of vitamin supplements to the diet, the expectant or nursing mother should determine her dosage under the direction and care of her physician.

Breast Feeding Vs. Bottle Feeding

It might be expected that while the new mother is still feeding her baby in the hospital doctors would prescribe the correct feeding methods along with vitamin dosage. Unfortunately many pediatricians are either indifferent to the baby's feeding or actively encourage bottle feeding. Although today's commercially produced infant formulas do an excellent job of duplicating the mother's milk, there is really no perfect substitute for breast feeding, provided the mother is in good health and does not suffer from nutritional deficiencies herself.

Not only does the baby benefit from the essential nutrients his mother's milk provides, but both mother and child are enriched by the closeness and mutually satisfying experience of nursing. It should be pointed out, however, that there are limitations on the value of breast feeding, such as that put forth in one of the leading textbooks on nutrition: "With an adequate supply of human milk most of the nutritional requirements of the newborn are met, except for iron and vitamin D. Breast feeding should, however, not be relied on exclusively for optimal nutrition beyond the first semester of life."

The controversy between breast feeding and bottle feeding continues, with the more advanced nutritionists advocating a return to the older practice of breast feeding, but the vital role of Vitamin E during the lactation period seems certain. An analysis of the vitamin's importance is provided by Bailey, who cites findings that show that cow's milk does not provide such elements essential to human nutrition as Vitamins E, A, and C, nicotinic acid, linoleic acid, fat, and iron. He cites Dr. F. C. Aitken of the Rowett Research Institute, Aberdeen, and Dr. F. E. Hytten, University of Aberdeen, whose joint research points toward the need of Vitamin E supplementation for babies "in order to prevent destruction of the infants' red blood cells." He states that Vitamin E and other nutritional supplements are "almost never added, because of the current medical faddism about extra vitamins being unnecessary, either for the pregnant mother or for the new-born or the premature, or the child or the adult, or the aging individual."

duced infant formulas do an excellent job of duplicating
the mother's milk, there is really no perfect substitute for
breast feeding, provided the mother is in good health and
does not suffer from nutritional deficiencies herself

Diets of Primitive People

Studies by sociologists and medical authorities show a strong connection between poor nutrition and the emotional ills of our society. Many of the tendencies toward unhappiness, alienation, violence, and other anti-social attitudes among both youth and adults can be traced back to infant and early childhood influences, including the comparative rarity of breast feeding. Lacking the closeness of the mother's body as their first emotional experience with the world, many people develop an insecurity and psychological instability that affect them throughout their lives.

The famous American anthropologist Margaret Mead is a strong advocate of breast feeding and advances it as one of the reasons why the peoples of the South Seas whom she studied are so much more happily adjusted to the communities in which they live.

The noted British surgeon Robert C. McCarrison, who served in the Gilgit area and lived for seven years among the Hunza peoples, remote in the Himalayas, made similar observations: "In Hunza, infants are reared as nature intended them to be . . . at the mother's breast. If this source of nourishment fails, they die; and at least they are spared the future of gastrointestinal disorders which often have their origin in the first bottle." It should be added that the Hunza people, who are noted for their longevity and general good health, enjoy a diet that is especially rich in natural sources of Vitamin E. Thus the Hunza mother passes this benefit on to her child. Infant mortality is practically unknown, in contrast to America. The adult Hunzakut was found to be physically healthier and emotionally more stable than the adult in our own country.

93

Dr. McCarrison also noted that in addition to an absence of heart and lung diseases, ulcers, cancer, kidney ailments, and other malfunctions, there was no insanity, no crime, no drug addiction or alcoholism, no problems of juvenile delinquency or sexual immorality.

The late Dr. Michael Walsh, who studied Indians in an isolated district in Mexico, found the same good physical, mental and community health. Similar conclusions were arrived at by Dr. Weston A. Price, who investigated the dietary habits not only of the South Sea peoples but also those in remote Alpine villages, the Isle of Man, the New Hebrides, Australia, and New Zealand, Central Africa, the South American jungles, and northern Canada and Alaska. Although their diets were largely confined to meat and fish, without vegetables or grain, or vegetables and grain, without meat or fish, they were in every case meeting the body's nutritional needs.

These same investigators found in villages only a few miles away, where Western man had brought white flour, white sugar, canned goods, and other processed foodstuffs, just about every disease that plagues "civilized" man.

The common denominator of the diets of these primitive peoples is that they tend to be rich in the natural sources of Vitamin E, as well as other nutrients. Our day-to-day nutritional problem is, of course, to adhere to a diet that is practical for the average American and that approximates the nutritional values found by the researches of Price, McCarrison, and Walsh without our having to limit ourselves to stone-ground grain or sun-dried apricots. It seems highly probable that the positive aspects of these primitive cultures result from their excellent nutrition, the benefits of which are passed on to the children through breast feeding. Ideally, then, American mothers should enrich their diets with Vitamin E and other vitamins and

should make an effort to breast feed their babies for as
long as they can.

Feeding Your Child

While breast feeding her baby and for a few
weeks after weaning, the mother's diet should continue
exactly as before and there should most emphatically be
no reduction in the intake of Vitamin E and other nutritional supplements. The need for Vitamin E is greatest
during the last four to five months of pregnancy and
throughout lactation. Although it varies with the individual
mother and child, the age of one month is usually considered the right time to begin giving the baby food in addition to milk.

Baby foods have been found to be deficient in Vitamin
E. Vitamin E is lost in baby cereals through the refining
process. Since it became known that babies are low in
Vitamin E and chemical analysis showed baby foods
lacked this vital substance, nutritionists have recommended
Vitamin E-rich foods and supplements. The Dick-Bushnell
report concluded: "These infant formulas and cereals had
such low levels of alpha-tocopherol that they might be
unsatisfactory sources of tocopherol for infant consumption. Supplementation of all infant formulas with alpha-
tocopherol is indicated."

Another cautioning factor about baby food is that,
although the relationship between salt intake and high
blood pressure has been known for years, the sodium
content of commercial baby foods has not been decreased,
and some doctors are still advising mothers to give them to
their babies. To get away from this practice, and to get
back to a more natural way of feeding babies, the mother
may decide to prepare her own infant's food herself. An

electric liquifier turns solid fresh meats and vegetables into a consistency a baby can manage with ease. The mother can thus use foods that contain their original nutrients, including Vitamin E, and that have not been salted and otherwise processed.

Today many mothers also try, whenever possible, to feed their families organically grown foods and meat that has not been subjected to chemical additives in feed or after slaughtering. What this is, of course, as in the case of the return to more extended breast feeding, is a shortcut around the food processing methods which have created an ever wider gap between rich and healthy soil and the final food products that reach our kitchens. Nothing could be more in need of such a back-to-nature movement than infant nutrition, which establishes the patterns of body chemistry for a lifetime.

X A Healthier Menopause

Many women spend their lives dreading the
menopause. Innumerable women believe that this is the
signal for them to retire from life. Others, who may have
read the reports of Kinsey, Masters and Johnson, or other
sex researchers, fear the onset of sexual appetites beyond
their previously established norms of intercourse. If they
first fear the cessation of sexual attraction and power, they
should look to the second for reassurance. Obviously, one
or the other of these fears has to be ill-founded.

Actually, sexual desire and the capacity of a woman
who has passed through the menopause is less controlled
by natural hesitations than it was when she was menstru-
ating. The timing of this new beginning in a woman's life
is usually related to the age at which menstruation first
began. Women who began to menstruate at eleven or
twelve often do not experience menopause until they are
in their fifties. Those whose periods began later—say at
eighteen or nineteen—may begin menopause in their
middle forties. The so-called little menopause, which may
be noted at ages thirty-eight to forty, is manifested in a
change of menstrual rhythm or flow. When it occurs, only
ignorance should allow it to cause concern.

Sexual Satisfaction and Health

Women should not confuse their menopause with their sexual maturity. It is not uncommon for a woman to acquire full sexual realization for the first time at thirty, forty, or even later. Some women have been taught so well that procreation is the basis of a woman's sex activity that they have learned to ignore the self-fulfilling aspects of sex. Sexual satisfaction is a matter of physical health and personal attainment; it is not related to age. The menopause, on the other hand, is entirely a function of age and of procreation and has nothing to do with the other aspects of sexual behavior.

During the menopause, the ovaries cease their production of hormones. This does not mean that these secretions disappear. During the fertile years, female sex hormones are produced at the rate of forty units of estrogen every twenty-four hours. During very advanced years—in the eighties and beyond—this figure may fall off to seven units in each twenty-four hour period. Other endocrine secretions which affect sex behavior are manufactured by the pituitary and adrenal glands. These glands show no significant change with the advance of years.

Menstruation and Vitamin E

When menstruation begins, it is especially vital that the young girl supplement her diet with large doses of Vitamin E, which should be continued until her periods are regularized. With normal menstruation during her reproductive years, a woman loses from 35 to 70 milliliters of blood per period, representing a total loss of iron in hemoglobin of 15 to 25 milligrams. Over the span of her reproductive years, the normal woman has a continuous loss of .5 to 1.0 milligrams of iron per day. Pregnancy deprives her still further, since the net iron loss during a full-term pregnancy has been conservatively estimated at 500 to 700 milligrams. Since without adequate replacement in a woman's diet she is in a precarious state of iron balance, iron supplements have become standard practice. Unfortunately many women do not realize that if the system is to replace blood losses with healthy blood, Vitamin E is as important as iron. Necessary as iron supplements are, by themselves they are not sufficient to insure healthy blood.

After the age of thirty many women experience their first menstrual irregularities. Doctors have reported that these excessive or scanty flows have been successfully regularized with Vitamin E. So too have been the numerous other difficulties that a woman in her thirties may experience. Dr. Henry A. Gozan reports that unusually high blood storage of estrogen can be reduced to a normal level and small blood vessels dilated so that concentration of the blood in the abdomen is lessened. He also reports a reduction of sweating and, with that, a lessening of strain on the sympathetic nervous system. Of sixty-six women he treated with Vitamin E who suffered from flushing, headaches and extreme nervousness, fifty-nine were completely relieved of these symptoms.

Relieving Menopausal Symptoms

Current medical opinion states that supplemental female sex hormones (estrogen) might be prescribed with advantage at the time of menopause, keeping women healthy and youthful during the middle years. If the prescribed dosage is small, menstruation will not recur.

The result will be an increase in bodily strength. Evidence, however, also indicates that Vitamin E, without hormone injections, may also help regulate hormones and provide the desired rejuvenation, without the side effects.

Many medical authorities recommend birth control pills or other female sex hormone tablets because this type of substitution therapy promises advantages, particularly for post menopausal women for whom a major cause of disability is bone fracture. An increase in skeletonal strength in the thin post menopausal bones would reduce the risk of injury.

This bone condition is known as osteoporosis and is believed to be due to the age-related decline in secretions of certain hormones by the sex and pituitary glands. No doubt other factors also contribute, such as lack of stimulating exercise and inadequate diet. The result is a decrease in bone-forming activity (ossification) with a consequent reduction in the amount of bone, although the composition of the bone remains normal. Manifestations include weakness, loss of appetite, hip and back pain, muscle tenderness and cramping, stooped posture, decreased height due to shrinkage of the spine, and a tendency of the bones to fracture easily.

Regarding menopausal ailments, Dr. Evan Shute writes: "One of the most generally recognized uses of alpha-tocopherol is for hot flashes and headaches at the change of life (menopause). Female sex hormone is the agent generally used for menopausal complaints, but too often this causes vaginal bleeding or 'spotting' which alarms the patient and her doctor; they may suspect cancer. Alpha-tocopherol never induces such spotting and is never in any way involved either in accelerating the growth of cancers already present or in initiating them. There is some suspicion that oestrogenic substances may. Alpha-tocopherol is usually not as effective as the latter for hot flashes; but it is often helpful, and its safety factor is strongly in its favour."

For many women hot flashes are frequently emotional in origin. They are rooted in a fear of unattractiveness and physical disability, common worries at the menopausal age. One of the indirect emotional benefits of using Vitamin E and maintaining a generally healthy diet and body is that these fears are avoided and faith in a worthwhile emotional future is kept.

Such changes as do occur in a woman's body following menopause, as we have noted, are almost entirely due to the reduction in the secretion of female sex hormones. There may be increased susceptibility to disease in the vaginal tissue plus a slight diminution in the size of the breasts. With the steady dietary supplement of Vitamin E, these changes are often so slight as to be unnoticeable.

Among the most common and annoying complaints at this critical time of life is an itching of the vulva and anus as the skin ages. A local application of Vitamin E in ointment form in addition to the oral dose will often bring relief. In acute cases, such treatments call for consultation and a physician's care and often, as Dr. Evan Shute notes, this use of Vitamin E requires "Very high dosage perhaps continued for long periods of time . . . and 4 to 6 weeks usually elapse before a response to treatment first appears. Often such a condition is the first warning of diabetes, and there, too, alpha-tocopheral is uniquely valuable, both for diabetic vulvitis and for other complications of that disease . . . Some women have local itching ascribed to discharge that persists long after the discharge has been cured. These women really have had two kinds of itching at once. Cure the one and the other comes to the fore. Alpha-tocopheral may help these people too, relieving the type of itching which has been unjustifiably ascribed to the 'discharge.' "

The use of Vitamin E during the menopausal period will help every woman keep her entire body in a healthier state. Unlike estrogen, Vitamin E will not change her mental attitudes or emotional states, but it will give her the more resilient body of youth and so provide the basis for a happy, worry-free maturity.

Many of the physical symptoms generally blamed on the menopause are caused by changes in the autonomic nervous system and are not directly related to the reduction of sex hormones. Flushing, palpitation, perspiration, and pounding of the heart are more often symptoms of general physical unfitness than of the menopause itself.

Women who have properly controlled their weight, kept their figures, and generally maintained their physical well-being will hardly understand what their friends are talking about when they recite their doleful catalogue of menopausal problems. Even mental and emotional problems are exacerbated by a lack of physical tone, caused usually by a lack of exercise, unnutritious foods, and a lack of sufficient Vitamin E supplements.

The world's foremost beauties, almost without exception, have kept their bodies in the highest possible state of health, if only to insure their attractiveness; and they have retained that attractiveness beyond what most of us regard as the normal term. They exercised, not only to retain their sex appeal, but to assure themselves of that emotional security which every woman needs. Such security cannot be felt by women whose physical condition is poor. Nevertheless, there are women who fear that too vigorous exercise will destroy their femininity. They are usually the women who also feel that proper dieting and vitamin intake is too much trouble, and that one must accept the physical decline of age as inevitable. A visit to the ballet should help to dispel both of those ideas. Not many ballerinas are created overnight. It takes many years of hard work and physical discipline to achieve stardom in the ballet, and dancers are usually rewarded by retaining their youthful vigor and appearance well into middle age.

Many women do not enjoy an active, happy sexual life during their young years. This may be because of their own upbringing or because of unsatisfactory contact with males. Nearly every physician is aware that this is much less true in the more mature woman, at least partly because fear of pregnancy has been removed. Biologically, many a woman is most a woman in her later years and far more of a complete person than she was during her youth. For the woman who has taken care of herself during her younger years, with proper exercises and by supplementing her diet with a healthy vitamin intake, there will be no need to feel those fears which beset many older women—that her romantic needs will be laughed at or seem absurd to others.

In fact, maturing women are apt to feel a greater need for romance in their lives as they advance in years. They will not achieve this unless they make a major bid for it through better health, and they should not expect to. But the woman who has learned to eat the right foods, supplementing them with the rejuvenating effects of Vitamin E, will give meaning to the lines of Robert Browning with her own life:

> "Grow old along with me!
> The best is yet to be,
> The last of life,
>   for which the first was made."

103

XI Is It a Fountain of Youth?

Juan Ponce de Leon, the sixteenth-century Spanish explorer, has gone down in history, less for his discovery of Florida than for his futile search for a fountain of youth. He had come to believe in a myth, an Indian legend that spoke of waters containing magical rejuvenating powers. If one studies the data on Vitamin E long enough, and in sufficient detail, one wonders whether all this information isn't just too good to be true. Is Vitamin E another fountain of youth, as elusive as Ponce de Leon's fantastic goal?

We have deliberately kept a good deal of the arguments about tocopherol out of the pages of this book, because they are simply not relevant to the clinical data. We are more concerned with causes and effects, with the results of experiments, with the validity of medical research papers, than with arguments about the acceptability of Vitamin E by this or that medical authority, on the pages of this or that medical journal.

But we cannot entirely ignore the controversy, because you must know about it in order to understand the role of Vitamin E in your own life.

104

Vitamin E and the Medical Establishment

We do not want you to see this vitamin, and the whole field of nutrition of which it is a part, as just another fad. Advertisements for various types of vitamins abound in nutrition magazines and health food stores feature Vitamin E prominently in their windows and on their shelves. What has caused this heightened interest? How legitimate is it? Will it go the way of other fads, from chlorophyll in toothpaste to Essence of Queen Bee in facial creams?

Is Vitamin E just another highly touted ingredient that eventually will wane in popularity, because people grow tired of it, because of newly discovered side effects, or simply because something has taken its place? These are important questions, to which every nutrition-conscious person must have answers. Vitamin E is not a phony fountain of youth. Arguments about it have become charged with attacks and counterattacks and some dealers have weakened its cause by pushing it indiscriminately in the manner of street vendors. But this would probably not have happened had not some sections of the medical profession systematically ignored and rejected Vitamin E. Because of this out-of-hand rejection, interest in the vitamin has worked like a jack-in-the-box; the more it is squelched the higher it rises.

For decades, the American Medical Association has been accused of ultraconservatism, of guarding the prestige—and pocketbook—of the medical practitioner with excessive zeal. Like most generalizations, this one is much too sweeping. The *Journal of the American Medical Association* may have failed to devote as much space to nutrition as we would like, but it does publish an enormous amount of valuable scientific information, and so do the journals of the state medical societies and the periodicals devoted to medical specialties. We live in a world of over-specialization, of tremendous work pressures on the individual physician, and so the layman must look out for himself, more than ever before.

You have to be your own medical guardian. You must be able to give your physician a concise and clear account of your health; and when the occasion arises you must ask him whether you may supplement your diet with vitamins, including Vitamin E. He may have reservations about other supplements, but if he is fairly well informed on the tocopherols, he may simply say, "Sure, it can't do you any harm." Better still, of course, if your physician is up-to-date on nutritional matters, he may prepare a diet supplement regimen for you, which will no doubt include Vitamin E.

The hullabaloo about Vitamin E is shared by other nutritional items, notably Vitamin C. This controversy reached a climax when Linus C. Pauling, the Nobel Prize-winner for chemistry, publicly advocated "massive doses" of Vitamin C, even in excess of 3,000 milligrams per day, to counteract the common cold. Among the criticisms of Dr. Pauling's advocacy were allegations that such high doses might well have undesirable side effects. It is difficult to call a Nobel Prizewinner a charlatan, but some of the critics came close to doing so. The issue is of interest inasmuch as Vitamin C and Vitamin E sometimes act in tandem, reinforcing each others effectiveness.

The Shutes and the Vitamin E
Controversy

Just as Dr. Pauling was the target for the Vitamin C critics, Drs. Wilfrid and Evan Shute have been the center of controversy concerning Vitamin E. These pioneers of tocopherol treatment have been ignored or denigrated for so long that they have grown sharp and bitter in their reactions. Dr. Wilfrid Shute has noted that heart attacks have been blamed on "stress and strain, on over-exertion, on the fast pace of modern living, on soft drinking water, on hard drinking water, and of course, on diets rich in animal fats." He notes that the chairman of the AMA's Diet-Heart Committee, who was scheduled to attend the Association's meeting in June 1967, had planned to outline dietary restrictions on animal fats during that meeting. But he was unable to attend because a coronary thrombosis had confined him to a hospital. Dr. Shute noted that this authority had for years followed a strict regime of low fat content in his food, coupled with regular exercise.

The Shutes often point out that the alleged causes of heart attacks were present in the lives of people prior to 1909 but did not cause coronaries. Dr. Wilfrid Shute finds "much evidence" that there is "no relationship between dietary fat and coronary artery disease." Instead, he maintains, the introduction of efficient milling methods in the manufacture of wheat flour have permitted "the complete stripping away of the highly perishable wheat germ," so that our diet has lost "its only significant source of Vitamin E." This change took place around the turn of the century, and coronary illness has been on the increase ever since. The Shutes are angry at organized medicine in the United States, and they are grateful that their residence in Canada has given them the freedom to research and publish that they feel would not be available in the United States. Nonetheless their ideas have gained wide circulation in United States periodicals and books, and the circle of those who are seriously investigating the uses and potentials of Vitamin E continues to grow in this country.

Versatility: a Double-Edged Sword

What does the Shutes' struggle for recognition of their work mean to you? As Wilfrid Shute has put it, "Other methods having failed, the time has come when the medical profession must adopt a method of proven success, basically sound, scientifically and abundantly verified by surgeons, physicians, and scientists the world over." Your own doctor may well be among those who have an open mind toward the challenges presented by Vitamin E and other nutrients that have substantial impact on human health or illness.

If one regrets the repressive or neglectful attitude that some members of the medical profession have displayed toward Vitamin E, the reverse jack-in-the-box effects are almost equally unfortunate. The remarkable versatility of the tocopherols has contributed to a general atmosphere of faddism and old-fashioned patent medicine hawking. Here, it would seem, is a cure-all! Anything wrong with your heart? Take Vitamin E. You've suffered a burn? Put Vitamin E on it. Pregnant? Take Vitamin E. Sexual fatigue? Vitamin E, of course. Dr. Evan Shute, in *The Heart and Vitamin E,* acknowledged that "no substance known to medicine has such a variety of healing properties" as Vitamin E, and that this very versatility has always been one of its major difficulties." It is simply "too useful for too many things." How could one seriously accept that the same substance that could help eliminate miscarriages might also remove scars in clawlike hands and be even more useful for diseases of the heart and blood vessels! Shute concludes that this "was asking too much."

The layman, who has seen his own share of highly touted cure-alls, with their almost inevitable side effects (include the scare about the birth control pill), cannot be blamed for doubting the multiple claims for Vitamin E. But the high-pressure mail-order catalogs and the flashy window displays should not distract us from the substantial proven values of the tocopherols. And the resentment of the Shutes is certainly an understandable reaction of two professional men who have devoted their lives to an apparently major medical development, but find themselves coolly dismissed by the American medical establishment.

Healthy Skepticism

Vitamin E has unusual properties in prevention and healing, and these include anti-aging factors. It is not a fountain of youth; it is not a cure-all; it may sometimes fail even in those areas in which its properties have been most firmly established. It acts in concert with other nutritional elements, and its multiple properties may at times be neutralized by environmental and hereditary factors. The advocates of Vitamin E, including the Shutes, naturally emphasize their successful experiences with the vitamin and tell us less about their failures. But we must assume that at times Vitamin E simply does not work. There are plenty of cases in which standard medical treatments do not bring about an improvement. And there are certainly nutritional methods that fail. Someone may report, not only in good faith but also with complete accuracy, "I've taken Vitamin C in large quantities before Pauling ever started to talk about it, and I still get a cold every winter!" No doubt, and if she did *not* get a cold, it might not even be due to Vitamin C. We are simply dealing with too many variables to be absolutely sure of the effectiveness of Vitamin E in every case and under every condition. There are no truly broad-based statistics available to show in how many comparative cases of, say, coronary danger, an actual thrombosis was avoided because of an intake of Vitamin E. Research statistics simply do not work that way.

Regardless of the many successful cases of Vitamin E treatment, the whole area of research is likely to remain a labyrinth of claims and counterclaims for some time to come. Writing in *Family Circle,* (August 1971), Ruth Winter noted that "until the full role of Vitamin E in the prevention and treatment of diseases is determined, enthusiasts are going to claim that it holds promise of helping practically every ailment under the sun." She added that even extravagant claims have some basis in fact, simply because Vitamin E contributes to the body's vitality which makes it more resistant to disease. Such caution, even in a mass magazine, is appropriate in the face of too much clamour on the one hand and stony silence or total rejection on the other hand.

A similar attitude should be adopted by the interested layman. Just because Vitamin E was cold-shouldered in the past does not excuse any present-day myth-making and legend-building; excessive expectations make for disappointments. Even if you are taking Vitamin E with your own physician's approval or guidance, you may still be unable to control your health to your full satisfaction.

110

And even if you are totally successful, you may never be sure that your improvement is specifically due to Vitamin E. The mature attitude in dealing with such still-evolving and controversial substances is one of optimistic but cautious expectation. Let yourself and your doctor be pleasantly surprised! If you go into your treatment without illusions, then you can't be disillusioned.

XII Vitamin E and Your Emotions

Over the past quarter of a century, medical science has directed increasing attention toward the effects of mental and emotional experiences on the body itself. More and more, doctors have come to realize that no clear line can be drawn between the mind and body. For instance, in many anxiety attacks there are both somatic manifestations—heart palpitation, disturbed breathing, tenseness, and muscle tremors—and emotional manifestations—the fear of dying, feelings of panic, and various indefinable fears. In more extreme cases there are also changes in heart rate, salivary secretion, gastric secretion, blood pressure and circulation.

A further interaction may be found between subjective sensory experience and observable changes in the electrical activity of the brain. In current research into the relation between emotions and brain action, notably the "biofeedback" technique, people have entered mental states enabling them to create alpha-wave rhythms in the brain and cause the waves to subside. With such extreme and sensitive influences being exerted by the mind on our bodies, it is not surprising to find, conversely, that the condition of our body has also been found to have an extensive effect on the well-being of the mind.

Research in both these areas reminds us that we are not a collection of unrelated parts, but a single, interrelated whole. Body and mind are so closely related that we cannot treat one without paying close attention to the other.

Effects of Vitamin E

It is not surprising to learn that Vitamin E has a large contribution to make in preserving a sound balance between the life of body and mind. But before dealing with specifics, let us review what we have learned about the major effects of Vitamin E:

(1) Because it reduces the amount of oxygen required by body tissues it is of use in treating gangrene, coronary and cerebral thrombosis, diabetes mellitus, arteriosclerosis, congenital heart disease, as well as threatened miscarriage, and all forms of emotional or physical strain that may create breathing problems.

(2) It helps to melt blood clots and thus is essential in the treatment of situations where thrombosis is a danger, during and after coronary infarctions, childbirth, and operations.

(3) It expands blood vessels and capillaries, where there may be an inadequate blood supply, thereby improving circulation and combating arteriosclerosis and thrombosis.

(4) It strengthens the walls of blood vessels and capillaries and so is useful in the treatment of nephritis, rheumatic fever, purpura, retinitis (inflammation of the retina), miscarriage, and the premature detachment of the placenta.

113

(5) By dilating capillaries, which bring blood and oxygen to the skin tissues, it contributes significantly to the treatment of burns, wounds, chronic ulcers, and some types of skin disease.

(6) As a further consequence of these actions, Vitamin E serves to impede the formation of scar tissue, internally and externally, and on some occasions to remove it; this is especially important in the treatment of certain heart diseases, where damage to the heart tissue may have occurred.

(7) It increases the number of healthy platelets in the bloodstream, essential in the *normal* blood clotting process, and so is of value in the treatment of thrombosis.

(8) In 25 percent of the diabetic cases which suffer from blood vessel problems in their extremities, such as the threat of gangrene, Vitamin E reduces the need for insulin.

(9) It regulates the metabolism of fats and proteins, and so has a profound effect on all the bodily processes.

Mental and Physical Health

Since the effects of Vitamin E are largely directed toward the blood and circulatory systems, and since the effects of fear, tension, and other psychosomatic ills are concentrated in the vital areas of the heart, brain, and lungs, it is not surprising that Vitamin E should help in making a person less vulnerable to these ills. Of course, a person with a healthy body will be less susceptible to emotional disturbances than a person with weak health. But whereas proper diet, exercise, and sufficient intake of other vitamins and nutrients will produce a general state of health, only Vitamin E works directly and powerfully upon the blood and its circulation.

The bloodstream is the central transportation system of the body. Whether emotional ills arise in the mind and create physical ills, or physiochemical inadequacies cause mental ills, the importance of healthy blood and a well-functioning circulatory system cannot be overemphasized. Exactly how Vitamin E offsets emotional disturbances based on physical causes is not yet known, but then, the whole area of psychosomatic medicine is insufficiently explored. Still, Vitamin E's ability to act directly upon conditions in the bloodstream and its supply of nutrients to the heart, brain, and lungs make it of great value in reducing the likelihood of these organs being affected by psychosomatic complications.

One of the clearest illustrations, as we have seen, of Vitamin E's effectiveness in this connection is with the patient suffering from hypertensive heart. However, the body-mind relationship is so subtle that the effects of Vitamin E, as well as other vitamins and nutrients, may well be presumed to go far beyond what we presently surmise.

One of our bodily functions is the production and consumption of chemical products. Our moods and actions affect the production of particular chemical substances appropriate to our feelings. But if our actions do not match those feelings—if we are inhibited from the expression of our anger, worry, or fear—those chemicals remain in our system unconsumed. If these chemical substances remain loose in our systems for long periods of time—if they accrete and multiply—we shall eventually suffer emotional damage and physical malfunction. The only way we can combat and neutralize these accumulated toxic threats is to maintain our physical health, especially of the heart and lungs, the two areas that are highly sensitive to psycho-

115

somatic illness. Since Vitamin E contributes to the health of the entire circulatory system, it is also important in preventing and relieving psychosomatic disorders related to that system.

Regarding our physical reactions to emotional upset, let us note some of the effects on the heart: When we are angry the heart feels taut. When fear becomes acute, blood pressure drops, the heartbeat is affected. These conditions can be registered electrically. The poisons that fear creates may be powerful enough to cause a victim's death. Suggestive death—for example, voodoo death brought on through the practices of witchcraft—is by no means unknown. Its victims are literally "scared to death." Some strokes are caused by cerebrovascular failure resulting from emotional causes. We recall the case of a teacher, who remarked on the death of a hypertense colleague who had died from cerebral thrombosis, that "he blew his brains out—from the inside." This teacher was also a very tense man; curiously enough, he died in exactly the same manner about a year later.

The Chemistry of Tension

Chronic fear, or anxiety, and its chemistry is different from that of an abnormal threat. In the latter case, the body produces its chemicals to match the degree of fear involved. These can be less than fatal in a single instance, but their accumulation can be dangerous. Longer lasting tensions, such as chronic fear, which cannot be discharged through the body's expression are voided through the mind; that is, through the autonomic nervous system and the hormones of the body. Continuous anxiety can be as deadly or more deadly over a long period of time as a single moment of terror.

When we can express our feelings and relieve emotional stress by permissible means—as for example, tears or convulsive laughter, violent exercise, or enjoyable partying —no harm ensues. Otherwise the body's only hope lies in its being sufficiently healthy to withstand the chemical products that emotional disturbances cause. It is best to lay our foundation of defense in advance; to make up our minds that a healthy heart and lungs and brain depend to a large measure upon our blood and circulation, and this in turn depends very largely upon whether we are getting sufficient Vitamin E.

An ounce of prevention is worth a pound of cure. Since we know that *all vitamins tend to prevent what they relieve,* and since Vitamin E has proven its worth in cases of coronary heart disease, which kills increasingly every year and is a major expression of psychosomatic ills— why should we not solve the problem before it arises?

Vitamin E and Headaches

The common headache often results from psychosomatic causes. In cases of persistent or recurrent headaches, which are often symptomatic of deep-lying illness, Vitamin E has frequently proved of value. The causes for the serious headache may be anything from a swelling of the blood vessels in the head to a brain tumor, abscess, or hemorrhage. The use of Vitamin E can ease the relationship between the causes and blood oxygen as a means of relief. Wade notes that a "unique benefit for easing headaches through Vitamin E may be that it preserves the oxygen in the blood for extended periods. This would mean more efficiency as blood is pumped through the blood vessels of the head. Vitamins E and C seem to work together to keep the blood vessels flexible, healthy and less subject to the painful disturbances."

Eyestrain is a major cause of headaches. In tests covering a ten-year period French researchers determined that Vitamin E helps in treating disorders of this type. With children as their patients, they noted that Vitamin E helped halt deterioration of the eye and in some cases contributed to improve vision. A check made on these same patients eight years later indicated that the effects of vitamin therapy were lasting.

Taking Things to Heart

Further evidence of the connection between poor nutrition and mental and emotional disturbances is the U.S. Army's list of six major reasons for rejection of volunteers and draftees. In the order of their importance they are: poor eyes, poor teeth, chronic heart disease, defects of the muscles and skeleton, venereal diseases, and mental and nervous disorders. With the exception of venereal disease, every one of these disorders can be either directly or indirectly affected by nutrition. We might also note that the five major deficiences in American food—calcium, riboflavin, ascorbic acid, thiamin, and alpha-tocopherol—are all closely related to these causes of draft rejection.

In the case of psychosomatic and other mental disorders, as well as in cases of chronic heart disease, which affected more than one out of twenty Army selectees, the nutritional factors most deeply involved were Vitamin E and thiamin (Vitamin B_1). Between them, they specifically affect three parts of the body: the cardiovascular system, the nervous system, and the digestive system.

Although thiamin is primarily related to the nervous

systems and the digestive systems the connection between Vitamin E and psychosomatic symptoms is very close. Fear, and the tension that it causes, are spontaneous. Small things can cause us to react with fear as easily as great. As Bertrand Russell very well stated it, "Our instinctive emotions are those we have inherited from a much more dangerous world and contain, therefore, a larger proportion of fear than they should." There is no way we can completely avoid fear and tension, and these emotions cause additional quantities of hormones, adrenaline and norepinephrine, to enter our heart and cause it to use up its oxygen supply at a faster than normal rate. If this condition endures too long or occurs too often portions of the heart muscle can die from lack of oxygen. However, Vitamin E can retard or prevent this from happening.

Along with insufficient Vitamin E, a lack of exercise greatly increases the threat of physical damage from fear and tension. The tone of the autonomic nervous system is also important. It determines our ability to resist our inner attacks upon ourselves.

The parts which comprise this nervous system are known as the sympathetic and the vagus nerves. In a person who is unfit, the sympathetic part of this system is paramount. In the healthy man, the vagus dominates. When the sympathetic system dominates, the tension of the fear-response is enhanced and the heart quickly exhausts its oxygen supply.

In addition to easily exhausting the oxygen from the heart, other related responses are involved for the man who lacks sufficient Vitamin E. Blood pressure may rise, often to dangerous levels, and as circulation decreases the skin may turn cold. To get "cold with fear" is an actual experience. Additionally, more sugar enters the bloodstream. Extra energy is thus made available and we tend to become indifferent to the body's warnings of fatigue.

119

Our breathing rate goes up as the cells of our body demand increased supplies of oxygen. The threat that our blood may form dangerous blood clots is enhanced. Most heart attacks are the result of blood clots. If in addition to insufficient Vitamin E, there is also a lack of thiamin, our digestion may also be impaired and we may suffer extreme abdominal discomfort.

Tension and fear may be controlled to some extent, although it is probably impossible and even undesirable to avoid them altogether. A complete avoidance of stress situations would probably nullify the creative challenge of daily living. Nevertheless, in our battle with dangerous emotions, we should call upon not merely our will power, which is largely a mental effort, but also upon the power of Vitamin E, which gives our heart and other vital organs a chance to contribute their share.

XIII Once Again, Those Clever Japanese!

Dr. Herman Kahn, Director of the Hudson Institute, speaks of the twenty-first century as "the Japanese century." We have all seen Japanese products, from transistors to textiles and from paper dolls to intricate electronic equipment, capture world markets. During the global economic crisis of 1971, the big tug-of-war was between the U.S. dollar and the Japanese yen. If one looks at the list of countries whose research and production have led the world during the past decades, one also finds the Japanese in the forefront of Vitamin E studies.

The most dramatic illustration of this trend was the Fourth International Symposium on Vitamin E which took place at Hakone, Japan, from September 7 to September 9, 1970. Participants came from the United States, Canada, Japan, West Germany, Switzerland, the Netherlands and Thailand. If the roster of researchers had been more complete, representatives from the Soviet Union, Hungary and Czechoslovakia would also have been present. This was the fourth such meeting. Earlier such conferences were held in 1939 in London, in 1949 in New York, and in Venice in 1955.

121

Japanese Research in Vitamin E

Other researchers were impressed by the pioneer work some of their Japanese colleagues had done. There are sound economic reasons for Japanese interest in Vitamin E research. The meeting at Lake Hakone, less than a hundred miles north of Tokyo, was sponsored by a commercial firm, the Es-ai Company. The company is presumably aware of the vast potential market for Vitamin E throughout the world, the limited production capacity in North America and Europe, and the ready availability of cereal grains on Japanese soil. Where there is a research-and-production gap in the West, Japan has consistently shown that it is willing and capable of filling it.

In other words, there is sound economic motivation for Japanese research on Vitamin E, and the papers presented at the Hakone congress gave evidence of a variety of studies being conducted on the relationship between Vitamin E and human health. A team of three Japanese researchers presented a study on the absorption of the vitamin into various parts of the human body. One specialist, Dr. H. Fukuba, reported on the ratio of Vitamin E in body fats; the study pointed up the different diet patterns in Japan and the United States. Participants also heard Dr. K. Kato speak of the presence or absence of Vitamin E in rats and show the vitamin's impact on liver functions.

Another research project dealing with liver health and performance was presented by Dr. K. Tanikaa. His paper, entitled "Effect of Vitamin E on ultrastructural changes of liver induced by alcohol" dealt with liver swelling "in acute alcoholic intoxication." Results showed that "Vitamin E may have a preventive effect" on the swelling of delicate liver parts caused by alcohol; it seems to reduce the accumulation of toxic elements in the liver. A related study, by Dr. A. Takada, on "The effect of antioxidants on liver injuries," concerned itself with the destruction of cells in the liver; the paper covered experiments with various agents, Vitamin E included, to see how such destruction takes place and may be prevented.

The impact of Vitamin E on iron deficiency anemia was noted by Dr. T. Fuji. His study, which used human adults as subjects, suggested that Vitamin E and iron may be taken in conjunction, both in their own way counteracting anemia. A related study, by Dr. T. Itoga, was based on clinical experiences with twenty women suffering from iron deficiency anemia. They were treated with iron and Vitamin E administered separately as well as together. A combination therapy was found superior to the use of either of them separately, perhaps caused by "a direct or indirect influence of Vitamin E on the metabolism of the bone marrow fat."

Maintaining Blood Quality

Blood stored for transfusion must retain its qualities, and medical research is constantly concerned with its stability in storage or transit. A paper by Dr. I. Kurokawa reviewed the "Effect of vitamin E upon the preservation of blood." He found "the preservative effect" of Vitamin E "comparatively good." Fragility of the skin in diabetics was tested by Dr. V. Hirata, who found that Vitamin E "actively strengthens the capillary resistance to negative pressure in some patients." A related paper by Dr. M. Kamimura showed that Vitamin E increases blood circulation through the veins of the skin, having "an

123

accelerating and normalizing effect" on "microcirculation in the human," particularly in the skin areas.

A major research project, in which eleven Japanese researchers participated, used a bloodless method of measuring pulse wave volume to establish the effect of Vitamin E on arteriosclerosis. They checked on the elasticity of the walls of arteries among 535 patients suffering from a variety of heart and artery illnesses. The research team reported that "the beneficial effect of Vitamin E on arteriosclerosis was proved quantitatively" by the pulse wave volume.

Other Research Experiments

The Hakone congress provided a forum for the most up-to-date reports on Vitamin E research, and it gave participants an opportunity to exchange information on work in progress. From Switzerland came a report by Dr. U. Gloor dealing with the absorption of Vitamin E. A visitor from the Netherlands, Dr. I. Molenaar, presented a paper dealing with the impact of Vitamin E in the blood on membranes of cells. Two teams of German researchers, each made up of two members, offered experimental results. Drs. V. and E. Bohlau were able to report on sixty thousand tests on healthy, sick, and convalescent persons. Their paper, entitled "Clinical investigations on the efficiency of the body under the influence of Vitamin E," concluded that "the recovery quotient improved, that the oxygen saturation of the blood increased, and that the fat metabolism was influenced positively in a number of patients." They indicated that Vitamin E treatment "can improve the physical capacity" of people in later life.

The second West German team, Drs. H. P. Hewing and

H. Hochrein, reported on work with thirty-nine patients suffering from heart ailments who had been given digitalis but had experienced "digitalis intoxication." Their symptoms included nausea, vomiting, diarrhea, and blurred or colored vision, or could be observed on their electrocardiograms. While each patient presented a special problem, the overall tenor of the Hewing-Hochrein report was that Vitamin E had hastened the patients' recoveries.

Among the participants from the United States were Drs. G. A. Emerson and J. S. Lewis, who reported on the Vitamin E level found in human blood during various stages of health in males and females from infancy to old age. Some were obese and some not; several subjects suffered from diabetes. The presentation provided wide background for future studies. Dr. C. Fitch reported on experiments with rhesus monkeys that showed that lack of Vitamin E resulted in anemia and muscular dystrophy. He found that "these manifestations of vitamin E deficiency may not become evident until one or two years after young monkeys are started on a purified diet, but thereafter the disease progresses rapidly to death within a few weeks." Dr. W. Reichel, also from the United States, reported on pigment changes in various parts of the body, including glands when Vitamin E is deficient. Experimenting with rats, he found that lack of the vitamin brought about conditions that were equivalent to premature aging. He suggested that "Vitamin E deficiency and senescence (aging) may share common mechanisms" within the body's functions.

Prevention—Not Cure

The congress at Hakone also heard Dr. Evan Shute who offered a brief history of Vitamin E studies.

He noted the resistance to Vitamin E research and therapy in many parts of the world, but said that "many vitamins beside Vitamin E have had a hard time getting acceptance, especially Vitamin C, but also Vitamin A and nicotinic acid, for example." He added: "It is difficult for medical authorities, once they have taken a stand, to reverse themselves. Then, too, nutrition is on the very fringe of medicine. There are very few courses on the subject in medical schools. Another difficulty is that doctors are taught to *cure* but not to *prevent* disease, and nutrition is really a parameter of prevention."

After noting that Vitamin E is "almost too useful," and "needed for too many reasons by too many people" to make its functions easily understood, Dr. Shute emphasized that the vitamin "is not so much cure as treatment." He said "it should be more widely emphasized that it is a prophylactic (preventive agent), and surely the future of medicine lies in prevention, not cure." He cautioned his listeners to be careful in the dosage of Vitamin E, particularly when treating chronic rheumatic heart disease. Dr. Shute said bluntly, "We believe that Vitamin E improperly used can kill." He concluded by saying that, looking back over the history of Vitamin E, "one is impressed by its versatility" and by "the fundamental role it plays which makes it helpful in so many pathological conditions."

XIV   Is Vitamin E Right for You?

By now you may be ready to go right out and buy large quantities of Vitamin E—because, no matter who you are, something in this book probably applies directly to your own health problem. But, as we have noted, the nutritional needs of no one person are identical with those of anyone else. And what may be just fine for your next door neighbor may be quite inappropriate for you.

Are you impatient with us? Are you telling us, under your breath, that we are pointing to the apparently highly useful potential of Vitamin E, while forever pulling our punches with ifs and buts? If you do, you are quite right. It is not your fault, nor is it ours, if the controversy about the whole field of nutrition leaves much to subjective judgment. On the one hand, major segments of the medical profession still ignore the importance of recent research in nutrition.

What's more, the courageous Doctors Shute themselves caution against two dangers: self-medication and wrong doses of Vitamin E. Theirs is the most well-informed, the most helpful, and ultimately the most meaningful advice.

Don't doctor yourself! Don't play a game of roulette with your dosage of Vitamin E!

We most definitely do not want you to treat the field of nutrition, the use of vitamins generally and that of Vitamin E in particular, as just another fad. It may well be that the whole area of Vitamin E therapy does not apply to you at all. Whatever your health problem, there may be entirely different alternatives to nutritional treatment.

Educating Your Physician—Tactfully

Then what are you to do?

You may well have to educate your own physician. Because of overspecialization and the scarcity of doctors, which results in many of our best doctors being terribly overworked, your own physician may find it difficult to keep up with the ever increasing quantity of information on nutrition. You should also try to understand the reluctance some doctors have toward nutritional therapy: its concept is relatively new, it has long been a province of charlatans, and it is full of unexplored areas.

How can you educate your own doctor? With tact, caution, questions, and with your own eagerness to learn from him. Try to inform yourself as much as possible about nutrition in general and Vitamin E in particular. But remember, in discussing these matters with your doctor, that you are a layman. Nothing infuriates a physician more than a patient's demands for a new drug or treatment he has read about in a popular magazine, usually under the heading "New Hope for . . . ." What the doctor knows, and you must learn too, is that these reports often deal with ongoing research on products so new that they have not yet been deemed safe or necessarily effective for general use.

Some aspects of nutrition and vitamin use are, relatively speaking, also still in an early stage of medical research.

But it is now really up to each physician to do his own more intensive reading on these subjects and not to permit himself to be isolated from what has become a mainstream of worldwide interest among searching medical men and alert laymen. Every one of us has to be the main guardian of his own health and that of his family and should try to integrate vitamin use into the overall pattern of health care. Doctors may disagree with us on the application of vitamin therapy, but they surely agree that the patient himself is the main protector of his health. They also agree that we must all become more active in practicing preventive medicine. That, certainly, is one area in which we can become more proficient, around which we can plan our daily lives to a much higher degree.

Vitamin E must be seen within the overall framework of a woman's or man's general life pattern. Thus, as you approach your physician, you are not just consulting him on Vitamin E but on the role this and other vitamins play in the general pattern of preventive medicine you are creating in your life. We know the negative effects of tobacco and alcohol, we know about the misuse of drugs; but it is now no longer enough to select things we must avoid. We must learn what, specifically, is really good for us.

Gently and carefully you must nudge your doctor toward telling you what he thinks is good for you. He may have done his own thinking on vitamins; he may have been caught up in the Vitamin C controversy, for instance; he may, for all you know, have been taking vitamins himself on an experimental basis.

But no matter how careful you want to be not to antagonize your doctor with laymen's naivete, in the end you are responsible for your own body and mind, for your own ultimate health—and concern for your doctor's feelings must give way to your health needs. You may have to switch doctors. There are now a great number of highly qualified physicians in this country who are deeply nutrition conscious. They could not care less what their professional organizations think about nutrition therapy, whether medical associations are burning Adelle Davis in effigy or simply ignoring the increasing public attention that nutritions studies enjoy today.

A nutrition-oriented physician is your best ally in practicing preventive medicine on yourself. You are probably aware of the detrimental chemicals that have crept into many of our foods, and you know much of what has to be avoided. But a personalized regimen of healthy foods, plus vitamins, is something that only a nutrition-oriented medical man—one who knows your health needs well—can prescribe. It is pointless to go on a Vitamin E binge, carried along by the information contained in this book. We don't want you to do anything of that sort. But we'd like nothing better than for you to find out, conclusively, that your normal food intake makes this or any other supplement unnecessary. If this should turn out to be true, you can count yourself very, very lucky. But it is unlikely.

The Mother: Guardian of Family Health

It is simply impossible to live a life in modern civilization without experiencing strain on its natural balance. Perhaps the most common strain is emotional rather than physical. Nutrition fits into the natural balance we all try to achieve and maintain—including, of course, sufficient sleep, some healthy exercise such as walking, weight control, and the avoidance of overexertion and stress of all kinds. With such a regimen, Vitamin E might well fit as an important link in the chain of living.

It is in this area that the role of the wife and mother

becomes crucial. In many ways, she is the physical and emotional "traffic cop" of the home. It is she who acts as a kindly buffer between the kids and the man of the house who has just returned home after a trying day downtown; it is she who must arrange the day so there is time for the trip to the orthodontist, the drive over to the community dance, the dinner with the new couple down the street. And it is she who must, with the skill of feminine family diplomacy, present nutritious food—and all that goes with it—to husband and youngsters with gentle firmness.

In a way, the mother is the family's foremost physician. Teachers cannot take the place of parents in the upbringing of boys and girls; and doctors—we have reluctantly come to realize—adopt more and more the role of technicians rather than guides and guardians of families. They can advise, they can caution, they can treat specific illnesses, but the day-to-day battle for survival is largely in the hands of the woman of the house.

Vitamins in Daily Living

This is not a bad thing, although it adds responsibility where there is already a good deal of it. Vitamin therapy is not the imposition of alien chemicals upon a family's food. Rather, it is part of daily living that makes allowance for the way in which the pattern of our lives has changed. We have begun to use air conditioning because of the heat and the deterioration of the air around us. But even that isn't very different from the way in which we have always controlled our environment with clothing, buildings, and heating.

Food has always been a means of therapy, whether it was applied to physical or emotional health. Each one of us has a favorite relaxing or refreshing food or drink, often associated with childhood pleasure. Symbols of nature, such as honey, have retained their emotional pull for most of us. Just because vitamins come as capsules, powders, or pills makes them no less a part of modern daily living. A Vitamin E pill is an aesthetically attractive item; golden, transparent, pearl-like. To find it next to one's plate might well become an attractive piece of decoration, part of the pattern in which a table is set. Our women's magazines do a marvelous job of teaching details of attractive living, and it is to their credit that they are taking an increasingly strong interest in the aspects of nutrition that are represented by vitamin therapy.

All these elements need to be combined for a sound program of family health: the choice of the physician who can act as an adviser on use of vitamins; the family living pattern that by now includes positive aspects of nutrition as a matter of course; the health-oriented life of parents and children in which preventive medicine includes nutritional values with rest, exercise, and harmonious living.

That is the key to true preventive medicine, of health awareness and creative therapy: harmonious living. It is into this pattern that a nutritional factor such as Vitamin E should be fitted—in the specific manner required by each individual, which vary from person to person and within each individual during the various periods of our lives.

Appendix

PRESENT KNOWLEDGE OF VITAMIN E
Oswald A. Roels, Ph.D.

The following paper was published by Dr. Roels in the volume entitled Present Knowledge in Nutrition *(Third Edition, 1967). This authoritative work is published periodically by The Nutrition Foundation, Inc., New York, N.Y., and it is reprinted here with the Foundation's permission. Dr. Roels's paper provides an overview of current medical findings and opinions concerning Vitamin E, evaluating available material cautiously but noting promising findings and the challenge they represent in current*

nutrition as well as to further research.

Vitamin E was discovered when male and female rats failed to reproduce normally on diets of purified fat, protein, carbohydrates, minerals, and the growth factors which were known in 1922. Addition of fresh lettuce, yeast, wheat, oats, milk fat, meat, or dried alfalfa restored normal reproductive capacity to the animals, and it was found that the restorative factor could be extracted from these foods with organic solvents. The compound was therefore classified as a fat soluble vitamin and called tocopherol.

During the past several decades, a series of compounds chemically related to vitamin E have been discovered: four naturally occurring tocopherols and their corresponding tocotrienols. All the compounds of the vitamin E series can be considered as derivatives of a hypothetical compound, 2-methyl-2-(4,8,12-trimethyltridecyl)-6-chromanol, or TOCOL:

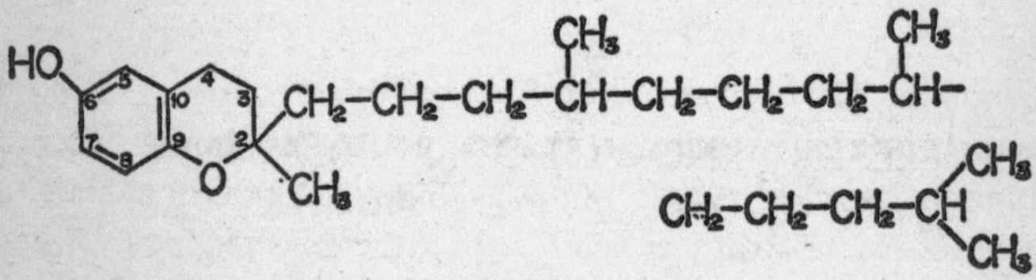

Alpha-tocopherol is 5,7,8-trimethyl tocol, *i.e.,* the derivative with methyl groups on carbon atoms 5, 7, and 8 of the ring. Beta-tocopherol is the 5,8-dimethyl tocol; gamma-tocopherol is the 7,8-dimethyl tocol; delta-tocopherol is the 8-methyl tocol; zeta 2-tocopherol is the 5,7,8-trimethyl tocol with additional double bonds between carbon atoms 3 and 4, 7 and 8, and 11 and 12 in the side chain or 5,7,8-trimethyl tocotrienol; eta-tocopherol is the 7,8-dimethyl tocol with double bonds between carbon atoms 3 and 4, 7 and 8, 11 and 12 in the side chain or 7,8-dimethyl tocotrienol; epsilon-tocopherol has been shown to be the 5,8-dimethyl tocol with double bonds in the same position in the side chain or 5,8-dimethyl tocotrienol; and delta-tocotrienol is the 8-methyl tocol with double bonds between carbon atoms 3 and 4, 7 and 8, and 11 and 12 in the side chain (J. Glover, in *Biochemistry of Quinones,* R. A. Morton, Editor, p. 248. Academic Press, New York, 1965).

134

At present, tocopherols are isolated on a commercial scale from vegetable oils, usually by molecular distillation, extraction with organic solvents, or absorption chromatography. Alpha-tocopherol is usually the most important homologue isolated from these sources; it can also be prepared synthetically.

Alpha-tocopherol absorbed from the intestine of cannulated rats appears in the animals' lymph, indicating a lymphatic route of absorption. Vitamin E is stored in the liver, and there appears to be a linear relationship between the amount of tocopherol in the diet and liver storage, although this may not hold for very high tocopherol intakes. Maximum storage occurs about six hours after administration of the vitamin. DL-Alpha-tocopherol acetate is absorbed much more slowly than the free alcohol. The bulk of the tocopherol stored in the liver cell appears to be associated with its structural parts, especially mitochondria and microsomes.

The relative biological activities of the tocopherol homologues vary greatly with chemical structure (J. Bunyan, D. McHale, J. Green, and S. Marcinkiewicz, *Brit. J. Nutrition* 15, 253 (1961)). Alpha-tocopherol is the most active biologically. Beta-tocopherol and alpha-tocotrienol have about one-third the activity of alpha-tocopherol and the other homologues exhibit relatively little biological activity.

S. R. Ames, M. I. Ludwig, D. R. Nelan, and C. D. Robeson (*Biochemistry* 2, 188 (1963)) found that the isomeric acetates of 2-L-alpha-tocopherol and DL-alpha-tocopherol were 21 and 60 per cent as active respectively as D-alpha-tocopherol acetate in the resorption-gestation rat bioassay. There was no evidence of a synergistic effect of the two isomers in this biological function. Subsequently, these relative activities have been essentially confirmed with other vitamin E deficiency conditions, including encephalomalacia in the chick and dystrophy in the chick, rat, and rabbit.

A review of the biological availability of various forms of vitamin E with respect to different indices of deficiency was recently published by B. Century and M. K. Horwitt (*Fed. Proc.* 24 *(4)*, *Part I, 906 (1965)*).

I. B. Desai, C. K. Barekh, and M. L. Scott (*Biochim. Biophys. Acta* 100, *280 (1965)*) have shown that absorption rates for D and L epimers of alpha-tocopherol acetate from intestines of normal and dystrophic chicks are similar. The Animal Research Council sub-committee for vitamin E standards has shown that the relative potency of D-alpha-tocopherol is 1.2 times greater than that of the DL-form.

Vitamin E deficiency causes a wide variety of symptoms in different species of animals, and may affect many different tissues: as already mentioned, reproductive ability is affected in both male and female rats. The female can conceive normally, but the fetus dies and is resorbed. In the male, there is a marked atrophy of the testes, frequently resulting in sterility. In turkeys and chickens, the adverse effect of vitamin E deficiency on reproduction is a high incidence of embryonic abnormalities and mortalities, resulting in low hatchability. The discovery that vitamin E was necessary to the house cricket *(Acheta domestica)* for normal spermatogenic activity and egg production indicates that alpha-tocopherol may be important for reproduction in widely different species.

One of the most widely occurring symptoms of vitamin E deficiency in many animals is muscular dystrophy. This has been observed in the dog, guinea pig, rabbit, chick, and *Rhesus* monkey. Whereas voluntary muscles are mainly affected in these animals, myocardial degeneration occurs in herbivorous animals.

In vitamin E deficiency, baby pigs suffer from degeneration of skeletal and cardiac muscle, degeneration of the liver, and creatinuria. Liver necrosis and muscular dystrophy do not occur in young fasting rats, but do occur in deficient rats on normal protein, low protein, or protein free diets. Nutritional muscular dystrophy also appears in infant lambs placed on a diet deficient in vitamin E. Fatal liver necrosis has developed in swine.

Neurological symptoms are observed in the chick suffering from vitamin E deficiency; encephalomalacia is common. The epithelium is also affected and massive exudative diathesis occurs.

Anemia has been observed, particularly in the *Rhesus* monkey. In this animal, skeletal muscle and bone marrow are most seriously affected. Increased erythrocyte fragility was a most significant hematological alteration in young mink deficient in alpha-tocopherol.

In human beings, it has been shown by F. Gerloczy and B. Bencze (*Acta Paediat. Hung.* 2, *4* (*1961*)) that sclerema neonatorum (a type of edema most common in the premature human infant) can be cured by oral administration of tocopheryl acetate; vitamin E therapy reduced mortality in this disease to one-seventh. The authors found extremely low levels of tocopherol in the serum of premature infants and ascribed the therapeutic activity of vitamin E to its influence on capillary fragility.

A. S. Majaj *et al.* (*Am. J. Clin. Nutrition* 12, *374* (*1963*)) have shown that Jordanian infants with severe kwashiorkor and macrocytic anemia and creatinuria showed positive improvement of the anemia following administration of tocopheryl phosphate and tocopheryl acetate. Urinary excretion of creatine decreased and there was a rapid increase in their reticulocytes followed by a rise in hematocrit, red blood cell count, and hemoglobin.

Horwitt (*Am. J. Clin. Nutrition 8, 451* (*1960*)) claims that alpha-tocopherol is important in the diet of man, and that the human requirement depends upon intake of unsaturated fatty acids. This claim was made as a result of a study on a group of adult male subjects who were put on a diet deficient in vitamin E for long periods of time. It was found that resistance of their erythrocytes to hemolysis, when incubated *in vitro* in the presence of hydrogen peroxide, was directly related to their dietary intake of alpha-tocopherol and inversely proportional to the polyunsaturated fatty acids in their diet.

It remains to be seen what is the physiological significance of decreased resistance to *in vitro* peroxide hemolysis of erythrocytes. As a result of these studies, Horwitt has recommended a daily intake of 5 mg. of alpha-tocopherol when the diet is low in unsaturated fat. When using high dietary levels of polyunsaturated fats, Horwitt recommends 30 mg. of alpha-tocopherol daily. It should be stressed here that the tocopherol content of natural oils and fats is usually proportional to their degree of unsaturation.

Very little is known about tocopherol excess in man. R. W. Hillman (*Am. J. Clin. Nutrition* 5, 597 (*1957*)) reported that a normal adult male ingested 296 g. alpha-tocopherol over a period of 93 days, with a resulting high level in his plasma (2.26 mg. per 100 ml.). A significant but transitory creatinuria occurred during the test period, but there was no apparent change in excretion of creatine or of 17-ketosteroids. The author could not detect any signs of clinical toxicity.

J. G. Bieri, L. Teets, B. Belavady, and E. L. Andrews (*Proc. Soc. Exp. Biol. Med.* 117, *131* (*1964*)) determined serum vitamin E levels in a normal adult urban population, and found no values below 0.5 mg. per 100 ml.; 6.1 per cent were below 0.7 mg. per 100 ml.; 70 per cent fell between 0.8 and 1.39 mg. per 100 ml., and 9.2 per cent were in the very high range. M. M. Rahman *et al.* (*Ibid.* 117, *133* (*1964*)) examined the serum vitamin E levels in a rural Pakistani population, utilizing exactly the same technique as Bieri *et al.* In this study, 21 per cent of the sample of the population examined was found to have serum alpha-tocopherol levels below 0.5 mg. per 100 ml., and 11.2 per cent of the sample had values below 0.4 mg. per 100 ml.

It is generally difficult to compare serum tocopherol levels reported from different areas because different methods are utilized by different workers, and many determinations of this compound may be unreliable. The analytical procedure is generally based upon a colorimetric reaction depending upon the oxido-reduction potential of the samples examined. Therefore, frequently total reducing substances are measured rather than alpha-tocopherol specifically. M. Y. Dju, K. E. Mason, and L. J. Filer, Jr. (*Am. J. Clin. Nutrition* 6, 50 (1958)) measured the tocopherol content of human tissues from birth to old age in necropsy samples of 70 individuals. They found that it was best to express tocopherol levels as milligrams of tocopherol per gram of fat rather than per gram of tissue.

Tocoperol levels in the lung, kidney, spleen and pancreas were of the same order as in the liver, skeletal muscle, and heart. In the pituitary, testes, and adrenals, however, levels were considerably higher. Wide variations were observed between individuals. The authors concluded that the difference in the tocopherol content of human tissues is largely caused by changes in dietary intake and absorption.

Although it is well known now that vitamin E is widely distributed in nature and that a deficiency causes a variety of symptoms in many species, its exact function at the molecular level in biological processes is not understood. Many workers have demonstrated that disease symptoms caused by its absence can be cured or prevented by a number of antioxidants. As a result, it has been suggested

139

that the sole function of alpha-tocopherol in biological systems is that of a lipid antioxidant preventing formation of peroxides from polyunsaturated fatty acids.

Thus, H. H. Draper *et al.* (*J. Nutrition* 84, 395 (*1964*)) found that when rats were fed a highly purified diet deficient in vitamin E the females did not reproduce. When the synthetic antioxidant N,N'-diphenyl-p-phenyl-enediamine (DPPD) was added to the diet at quite low levels, their normal reproductive capacity was restored. Bieri (*Biochem. Pharmacol.* 13, 1465 (*1964*)) demonstrated that several synthetic antioxidants, fed to chicks at relatively high levels, were ineffective in preventing exudative diathesis and mortality when the diet was deficient in both selenium and vitamin E. However, when either selenite or alpha-tocopherol acetate was given with the antioxidants, deficiency signs and mortality were prevented, indicating that there is a synergistic effect between antioxidants and selenium or vitamin E.

It had been demonstrated earlier that the onset of symptoms of vitamin E deficiency in the chick could be accelerated by increasing the polyunsaturated fatty acids in the diet, and that vitamin E deficiency could be delayed in the same animal by adding some known antioxidants. Addition of DPPD does not have a sparing effect on tocopherol stored in the liver of growing rabbits and rats fed a diet deficient in vitamin E. It has also been reported that ascorbic acid protects chicks from the characteristic lesions of vitamin E deficiency, even when they receive high dietary levels of polyunsaturated fats.

F. Christensen, H. Dam, and R. A. Gortner (*Acta Physiol. Scandinav.* 36, 82, 87, 97 (*1956*)) believe that alpha-tocopherol may be more than just an antioxidant; synthetic antioxidants could prevent some symptoms of vitamin E deficiency in the rat and chicken, but not others. Thus, certain antioxidants could prevent encephalomalacia but not muscular degeneration in the chick. Another anti-oxident could prevent muscular dystrophy but not encephalomalacia.

Interesting observations on the physiological role of vitamin E have come from J. S. Dinning, P. L. Day, and C. D. Fitch (*see Nutrition Reviews* 21, *289* (*1963*)). These workers have studied the *Rhesus* monkey fed a diet free of tocopherol over long periods of time. They found muscular dystrophy, creatinuria, anemia, and various other hematological symptoms in their deficient animals. Pathologic lesions of skeletal muscle and bone marrow were obvious. All these symptoms could be cured and reversed by feeding alpha-tocopheryl acetate or phosphate, whereas DPPD caused only partial reversal.

The 6-chromanol of hexahydro coenzyme Q_4 also reversed all symptoms of alpha-tocopherol deficiency. The same compound cures muscular dystrophy induced in the rabbit by a diet deficient in vitamin E. The possibility remains that the preventive effect of synthetic antioxidants may result from the antioxidant protection afforded the residual stores of alpha-tocopherol. Moreover, "peroxide" levels reported in different tissues of animals deficient in vitamin E may well have been manipulative artifacts.

A series of reports has appeared from K. Schwarz and co-workers (Schwarz and C. M. Foltz, *Fed. Proc.* 19, *421* (*1960*)) indicating that there is a complex physiological link between selenium and alpha-tocopherol. Both substances prevent exudative diathesis in the chick, but selenium does not prevent muscular dystrophy of rabbits on a diet deficient in vitamin E, nor will it prevent resorption gestation in rats. Schwarz *et al.* therefore conclude that a first group of diseases is due principally to vitamin E deficiency and may not be influenced by selenium. A second group is caused principally by selenium deficiency and is only partially affected by vitamin E, while still a third group is caused by a simultaneous lack of vitamin E and selenium: *e.g.* dietary liver necrosis in rats and multiple necrosis in the mouse.

This story was further complicated when it was shown that in certain cases amino acids containing sulfur have a sparing effect on vitamin E. It has been suggested that this is due to a possible contamination of the amino acids with selenium. However, Scott and C. C. Calvert (*J. Nutrition 77, 105 (1962)*)) indicated that, when chicks were fed a diet deficient in vitamin E, low dietary levels of methionine and cysteine accelerated the onset of nutritional muscular dystrophy. Adequate levels of L-cystine prevented muscular dystrophy.

A review of the biochemistry of vitamin E was published by F. D. Vasington, S. M. Reichert, and A. Nason (*Vitamins and Hormones 18,43 (1960)*)) and an excellent series of review papers on vitamin E appeared in *Vitamins and Hormones* 20 (*1962*).

Since vitamin E deficiency gives rise to nutritional muscular dystrophy in many species of animals, there have been intensive investigations of the effect of alpha-tocopherol on oxidative enzyme systems. As early as 1956, J. Bouman and E. C. Slater (*Nature 177, 1181 (1956)*; *Biochim. Biophys. Acta 26, 624 (1957)*)) reported the presence of alpha-tocopherol in active respiratory enzyme systems of heart-muscle preparation. Vasington and Nason (*Vitamins and Hormones, loc. cit.*) detected tocopherol in bovine heart NADH-cytochrome c reductase.

It was concluded from this that tocopherol may play a role in biological oxidation-reduction reactions. Indeed, Nason and I. R. Lehman (*J. Biol. Chem. 222, 511 (1956)*)) found a twofold to sixfold increase of NADH oxidation when alpha-tocopherol was added to partially purified particulate preparations of rat skeletal muscle; this increase was due to a restoration of cytochrome c reductase activity.

A. L. Tappel (*see Nutrition Reviews* 21, *23* (*1963*)) has demonstrated that muscular dystrophy in rabbits deficient in vitamin E may well be due to an increased fragility of lysosomes in the affected tissues. He observed that muscle degeneration was accompanied by an increased release of a wide variety of acid hydrolases from lysosomes. These hydrolytic enzymes act on their respective substrates and cause a general breakdown of nucleic acids, proteins, carbohydrates, mucopolysaccharides, and other cell constituents. This leads to typical muscular dystrophy.

A. Guha and O. A. Roels (*Biochim. Biophys. Acta* 111, *364* (*1965*); Roels, M. Trout, and Guha, *Biochem. J.* 97, *252* (*1965*)) have shown that, in vitamin A deficiency, increasing doses of dietary alpha-tocopherol increase the stability of the rat liver lysosomal membrane. J. A. Lucy and J. T. Dingle (*Nature* 204, *156* (*1964*)) have similarly demonstrated that alpha-tocopherol counteracts the lysis of rabbit erythrocytes induced by vitamin A during *in vitro* incubation.

It therefore appears that vitamin E plays an important role in insuring the stability and integrity of biological membranes. Whether this function is or is not related to its antioxidant properties remains to be seen.

Selected Bibliography

The following list of books, articles, and scholarly papers should serve two purposes: as a guide to sources cited in this volume, and as a basis for further reading on Vitamin E and related subjects. Although the literature in this field, notably in academic journals, has grown rapidly in recent years, the number of books addressed either to specialists or the general public remains limited. It is therefore necessary to study the specialized journals for current information.

The most complete guide to contemporary writings is the *Bibliography of Vitamin E*, published by Distillation Product Industries, Rochester, New York, a division of the Eastman Kodak Company. Seven volumes of this bibliography have been issued. Of these, the most recent, Volume VII (1965–1967) was published in 1968. The listing was compiled by Miss Wilma F. Kujawski of the Research Laboratories of DPI. In his preface to the Bibliography, Norris Embree, Vice President, Manufacturing and Research of DPI, notes that the large number of published papers "shows that scientists continued their interest in all aspects" of Vitamin E and are increasingly aware of "the intricacies of the interrelationship of Vitamin E with other environmental factors." Although this most recent volume of the bibliography covers only three years, it contains 1,500 entries.

In preparing *The Truth About Vitamin E,* we relied substantially on a unique periodical, *The Summary,* issued by The Shute Foundation for Medical Research, London, Ontario, Canada. The 1971 issue of this annual is Volume 23. The editor, Dr. Evan Shute, publishes abstracts of works dealing with Vitamin E from periodicals throughout the world, and often appends comments to these abstracts.

Recent references to Vitamin E may also be found in relevant general abstracts, such as *Chemical Abstracts, Biological Abstracts,* the *Index Medicus,* and the *Bibliography of Agriculture.*

Airola, Paavo. *Health Secrets from Europe.* Englewood Cliffs, N.J.: Parker Publishing Company, 1970.

Bailey, Herbert. *The Vitamin Pioneers.* Emmaus, Pa., Rodale Press, 1968.

———. *Vitamin E: Your Key to a Healthy Heart.* New York: Arc Books, 1970.

Bayer, R. "Results of Pretreatment with Vitamin E for Control of Primary and Secondary Essential Infertility." *Wiener Medizinische Wochenschrift,* Vol. 109, p. 271, 1959.

Beckman, R. "Results of Experiments on the Vitamin E Content of Human Milk and of Cow's Milk in Its Use in Pediatrics." *Milchwissenschaft,* Vol. 9, p. 365, 1954.

Bellet, S., et al. "Comparative Human Study: Coffee Linked to Fatty Acid Increase." *Journal of the American Medical Association,* Vol. 197, p. 197, 1966.

Binder, H. J., et al. "Tocopherol Deficiency in Man." *New England Journal of Medicine,* Vol. 273, pp. 1289–1297, 1965.

Borsook, Henry. *Vitamins.* New York: Pyramid Brooks, 1970.

Bortz, Edward L. *Creative Aging.* (C. E.: Author will provide additional info.)

Brewer, T. H. *Metabolic Toxemia of Late Pregnancy*. Springfield, Ill.: Charles C Thomas, 1966.

British Journal of Nutrition. A series of papers on "Vitamin E and Stress," Volume 21, 1967.

Brubacher, G. "On the Vitamin Content of Some Foods." *Internationale Zeitschrift für Vitaminforschung*, Vol. 36. pp. 409–415, 1966.

Call, M., and Lorentzen, D. "Rupture of the Liver Associated with Toxemia." *Obstetrics and Gynecology*, Vol. 25, p. 466, 1965.

Century, B., et al. "Biological Availabilty of Various Forms of Vitamin E with Respect to Different Indices of Deficiency." *Federation Proceedings*, Vol. 24, pp. 906–911, 1965.

Cheraskin, E., and Ringsdorf, Jr., W. M. "Daily Vitamin E Consumption and Reported Cardiovascular Findings." *Nutrition Report International*, August, 1970.

Cooper, L. F., et al. *Nutrition in Health and Disease*, 14th ed. Philadelphia: J. B. Lippincott, 1963.

Dahl, L. K. "Rose of Dietary Sodium in Essential Hypertension." *Journal of the American Dietetic Association*, Vol. 34, p. 585, 1958.

Dam, H. "The Role of Vitamin E in Nutrition." *Naeringsforskning*, Vol. 8, pp. 43–52, 1964.

Darby, W. J. "Tocopherol-Responsive Anemias in Men." *Vitamins and Hormones*, Vol. 26, pp. 685–701.

Davis, Adelle. *Let's Eat Right to Keep Fit*. New York: Harcourt, 1970.

Fiala, J., et al. "Preservation of Blood by Use of Vitamin E." *Vnitrni Lekarstvi*, Vol. 16, pp. 359–368, 1970.

"The Fountain of Youth in Your Kitchen." *Prevention*, April, 1971, p. 125.

"First Statistical Evidence: Heart Needs Vitamin E." *Prevention*, March, 1971.

Geller, L. "Vitamins in Cosmetics." *Seifen-Öle-Fette-Wachse*, Vol. 91, p. 412, 1965.

Gloor, U., et al. "Metabolism of Tocopherol." *Wissenschaftliche Veröffentlichung der Deutschen Gesellschaft für Ernährung*, Vol. 12, pp. 66–79, 1967.

Gordon, H. H. "Tocopherol Deficiency in Infants and Children with Steatorrhea." *Transactions of the*

American Clinical and Climatological Association, Vol. 68, p. 155, 1956.

Green, J. "Interrelations Between Vitamin A and E." Experimental Eye Research, Vol. 3, pp. 388–391, 1964.

Grollman, A., et al. "Sodium Restriction in the Diet for Hypertension." Journal of the American Medical Association, Vol. 129, p. 533, 1945.

Hastings, Donald W. A Doctor Speaks on Sexual Expression in Marriage. Boston: Little, Brown, 1966.

Herting, D. C. "Perspective on Vitamin E." American Journal of Clinical Nutrition, Vol. 19, pp. 210–218, 1966.

——————, and Drury, E. J. E. "Vitamin Content in Milk," American Journal of Clinical Nutrition, Vol. 22, pp. 147–158, 1969.

Horne, Jr., H. W., and Maddock, C. L. "Vitamin A Therapy in Oligospermia." Fertility and Sterility, Vol. 38, p. 231, 1952.

Jankelson, O. M., et al. "The Effect of Glucose Tolerance and Circulating Insulin in Men with Maturity-Onset Diabetes." Lancet, Vol. 1, p. 527, 1967.

Kempner, W. "Rice Diet in the Treatment of Hypertension and Vascular Diseases." North Carolina Medical Journal, Vol. 5, p. 125, 1944; and, Vol. 6, p. 62, 1945.

Koch, E. "Does a Clinical Vitamin E Deficiency Occur in Humans?" Ernährungswirtschaft, Vol. 11, p. 784, 1966.

Lepeshinskaya, Olga. Life, Age and Longevity. (C.E.: Author will supply additional info.)

Loutit, R. T. "Chemical Facilitation of Intelligence Among the Mentally Retarded." American Journal of Mental Deficiency, Vol. 69, pp. 495–501, 1965.

Lindner, E. "Therapeutic Value of Vitamin E in Disturbances of Spermatogenesis." Internationale Zeitschrift für Vitaminforschung, Vol. 29, p. 33, 1958.

McCullagh, E. Perry, et al. "A Study of Diet Blood Lipids and Vascular Disease in Trappist Monks." New England Journal of Medicine, Vol. 263, p. 569, 1960.

McDonald, P., Edwards, R.A., and Greenholgh, J. F. D. Animal Nutrition. Edinburgh, Oliver and Boyd, 1966.

Maqueo, M., et al. "Nutritional Status and Liver Function in Toxemia of Pregnancy." *Obstetrics and Gynecology*, Vol. 23, p. 222, 1964.

Martius, C. "Biological Action Mechanisms of Tocopherol." *Wissenschaftliche Veröffentlichung* der Deutschen Gesellschaft für Ernährung, Vol. 16, pp. 31–36, 1967.

Mayer, J. "Obesity and Cardiovascular Disease." *Journal of the American Dietetic Association*, Vol. 52, p. 13, 1968.

——————. "Hypertension, Salt Intake, and the Infant." *Postgraduate Medicine*, Vol. 45, p. 229, 1969.

Mengert, W. F. and Tweedie, J. A. "Acute Vasospastic Toxemia: Therapeutic Nihilism." *Obstetrics and Gynecology*, Vol. 24, p. 662, 1964.

Olson, J. A. "The Metabolism of Vitamin E." *Pharmacological Review*, Vol. 19, pp. 559–596, 1967.

Paddock, C. E. "Diet in Pregnancy." *Surgery, Gynecology and Obstetrics*, Vol. 31, p. 71, 1920.

Pharmacopoeia of the U.S.A., Philadelphia: Mack Printing Co., 17th ed., 1965.

Plate, W. P. "Recent Insights into the Problem of the So-Called Habitual Abortion." *Wiener Klinische Wochenschrift*, Vol. 77, pp. 798–802, 1965.

Price, Weston A. *Nutrition and Physical Degeneration*. Monrovia, Calif.: Price-Pottenger Foundation, 1969.

Raoul, Y. "The Transport of Vitamins in the Blood." *West European Symposium on Clinical Chemistry*, Vol. 5, pp. 99–119, 1966.

Roels, O. A., et al. "The Effect of Vitamins A and E on Biological Membranes." *Abstracts, Siebenter Internationaler Ernährungskongress*, Hamburg, Germany, 1966.

Second National Conference on Cardiovascular Diseases. *Report*. Washington, D.C.: U. S. Government Printing Office, 1965.

Shimazono, N., et al. "Fourth International Symposium on Vitamin E." *The Summary*, Vol. 22, pp. 2–15, 1970.

Shute, Evan. *The Heart and Vitamin E*. London, Ontario, Canada: The Shute Foundation for Medical Research, 1969.

Shute, Wilfrid E., and Taub, Harald. *Vitamin E for Ailing*

and Healthy Hearts. New York: Pyramid House, 1969.

Tani, M., et al. "Prevention and Therapy of Diabetic Retinopathy." *Saishin Igaku,* Vol. 19, pp. 2071–2078, 1964.

"Tocopherol Requirements in Infancy." *Nutrition Reviews,* Vol. 22, pp. 132–134, 1964.

Toverud, G. "The Influence of Nutrition on the Course of Pregnancy." *Milbank Memorial Fund Quarterly,* Vol. 28, p. 7, 1950.

Taylor, Renee. *Hunza Health Secrets*. Englewood Cliffs, N.J.: Prentice-Hall, 1964.

"Vitamin E." *Drug and Cosmetic Industry*. Vol. 97, p. 102, 1965.

"Vitamins That Protect Your Lungs." *Prevention:* December, 1970.

Wade, Carlson. *The Rejuvenation Vitamin*. New York: Award Books, 1970.

Weiser, H., and Weber, F. "Vitamin E Requirement." *Ernährungswirtschaft,* Vol. 11, p. 784, 1966.

Williams, J. W. *Obstetrics,* 13th ed. New York: Appleton, 1966.

Zierler, K. L. et al. "Report on the Effect of Vitamin E in the Treatment of Thrombosis." *American Journal of Physiology,* Vol. 153, p. 127.

Index

153